Testosterone Resistance

Testosterone Resistance

Fighting for the Men's Health Hormone

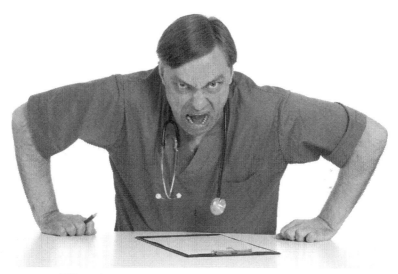

'What do you mean by the word NO Doctor?'

Malcolm Carruthers, MD

To order additional copies of this book, contact:
Xlibris
800-056-3182
www.Xlibrispublishing.co.uk
Orders@Xlibrispublishing.co.uk
738130

Dedication

To patients who have taught me so much about the benefits of testosterone treatment and to friends and colleagues who have supported me in the fight for testosterone replacement treatment (TRT), especially Mark Feneley, Professor Tom Trinick, Dr Adrian Zentner, Professor Ralph Martins, Professor Bruno Lunenfeld, Professor Svetlana Kalinchenko, Professor Abdul Traish, Professor Abe Morgentaler, and many others round the world. My sons, Andrew and Robert, also had valuable comments on the manuscript.

To my late friend Hugh Welford, good friend and ace computer programmer, who made my research possible.

The publication team at Xlibris, including especially Ada Tan, Jade Allen and Ace Sanchez, have been endlessly helpful in bringing the book together.

Last but not least, to my wife, Jean Coleman, Secretary and Cofounder of the Andropause Society, who has constantly supported me over the last thirty years and helped me sustain and survive the fight for the male hormone.

First they ignore you, then they laugh at you,
then they fight you, then you win.

Gandhi

Contents

Disclaimer

This book has been written purely from the belief that millions of men worldwide are being denied the many benefits of testosterone treatment because of the multiple influences discussed in this book.

No, I am not in the pay of that popular ogre Big Pharma or funded by other commercial organizations. I am a medical consultant to the Centre for Men's Health, a company running clinics in London's Harley Street, Manchester, and Edinburgh, but do not have shares in it. I am still in clinical practice part-time but am not financially dependent on it. I look forward to seeing testosterone replacement therapy (TRT) becoming an accepted part of NHS General Practice and continuing to argue the case for a more liberal view of TRT.

The costs of publishing and promoting this book have been paid for entirely by me, and any profits from this book will be donated to a registered charity established in 2000, the Society for the Study of Androgen Deficiency (Andropause Society).

I have never let my views influence my research findings and deny any conflict of interest.

Foreword

Foreword: Prof. Abe Morgentaler

Recently, I saw an eighty-three-year-old patient of mine for his annual office visit. He had been treated with testosterone for more than fifteen years. 'I'm doing great,' he reported to me. 'I still play tennis three times each week, and I have sex every week or two. When I compare myself to my contemporaries, many of whom are already dead or don't look so good, I feel as if testosterone has given me a secret advantage!'

This patient's story is commonplace among men with testosterone deficiency who have been treated with testosterone therapy. Although it is unfair to label testosterone as the fountain of youth or a panacea, every medical practitioner with experience with this treatment has seen cases of remarkable improvement in their patients in a variety of areas, including sexuality, vigor, mood, physical strength and appearance, and sense of well-being.

Indeed, these dramatic improvements have made me wonder whether this is all a placebo effect when I have first begun offering the treatment. However, I have quickly discovered that when men complain that the benefits have mysteriously disappeared, their blood levels of testosterone are low again. It is impossible for men to know this without a blood test—the effect couldn't have been a placebo. Men can tell when their levels are good, and they can tell when their levels are low. This is a real effect.

Unfortunately, as more and more patients and physicians learn about the benefits of testosterone therapy, there also arises a vocal antitestosterone community that has become enamored of any piece of evidence that may suggest a negative twist on the testosterone story. Today, testosterone therapy is arguably the single most controversial medical topic. It has been politicized to a degree that does not exist for any other medical treatment. And like any story that has captured the media's attention, the messages have become oversimplified, and outrageous comments are highly valued, regardless of their scientific merit. The consequences of this politicization are substantial, as physicians and the public have both been taught to fear testosterone therapy, despite its great therapeutic value and very reasonable safety profile.

Prof. Malcolm Carruthers has been a clear-sighted champion of testosterone from long before it became a fashionable concept. His experience and insight in the topic are formidable, and he writes in a style that is both incisive and entertaining. It is likely that every medical field has its unscientific assumptions and lore, but the field of testosterone deficiency and treatment has more than its share. Whereas many experts bow to the false god of assumed truths without questioning their wisdom or scientific provenance, Dr. Carruthers skillfully skewers many of these concepts. There is no one quite like Malcolm Carruthers, MD, and there is no other book quite like this one when it comes to describing the unvarnished truths about testosterone.

In October 2015, I chaired an international expert consensus panel on testosterone therapy, with participants from eleven countries on four continents, with a broad range of expertise that included endocrinology, urology, diabetes, general medicine, and basic science. We gathered to address many of the controversial issues discussed in this book and arrived at a set of statements that we expect to soon be published. Based on the best available evidence, the panel affirmed the high prevalence of testosterone deficiency among adult men throughout the world, the substantial negative impact of testosterone deficiency on the health and well-being of affected men, and the strong evidence in support of benefits of treatment and rejected the frequent assertions that testosterone therapy increases risks of prostate cancer and cardiovascular disease. Dr. Carruthers comes to the same conclusions but writes about them with freedom and singular entertaining style that academic writing can never achieve.

Testosterone deficiency is real, and the treatment often provides remarkable benefits, as noted in my eighty-three-year-old patient above. This book will not only open the readers' eyes to the medical underpinnings of the issues but will also explain why there is so much unnecessary controversy surrounding testosterone.

Abraham Morgentaler, MD, FACS

Founder and Director, Men's Health Boston

Associate Clinical Professor of Urology

Harvard Medical School

www.menshealthboston.com

Introduction:
A Lifetime of Testosterone Treatment

There is a backlash against testosterone treatment by the medical establishment and allied forces, which can be called external resistance, as well as the original idea presented here of internal resistance to the hormone in the body.

The argument of the external resistance forces goes: Because of heavy marketing by pharmaceutical companies that make testosterone preparations, sales, which were stable for years, have risen more than 1,800 percent in the United States, exceeding $1.9 billion in 2012. If, like most authorities, you define *testosterone deficiency* as a blood level below a certain value, then the frequency of the condition has not changed much over that period. There you are, they say. As they define it, the increased sales of the hormone is due to marketing hype and disease-mongering, and it is medically unnecessary, dangerous, and must be curtailed.

However, if you define it as a set of symptoms which gives you an identikit picture of the condition, then the number of patients who are aware of the disorder and try, usually without success, to convince their doctors to give them a trial of testosterone treatment, has increased by that amount or more. These symptoms include loss of libido, erection problems (particularly loss of morning erections), loss of energy, feeling of suddenly growing old, memory loss, depression, irritability, joint pains, and night sweats. They have been recognized as being associated with insufficient testosterone for over seventy years and are now being linked to several serious and increasingly common medical conditions such as diabetes and obesity.

If these characteristic symptoms then go away and stay away with a course of testosterone treatment and return when it's stopped, it is not just aging, and patients naturally want to stay on the treatment.[1]

However, lab test-obsessed doctors will demand low testosterone levels as well even if, as shown in many research studies, including my own practical experience in treating more than 2,500 patients over twenty-five years, these levels bear no relation to the symptoms except when they are very low. This simple but effective approach is on the basis of the old saying that 'if it looks like a duck, walks like a duck, and quacks like a duck, it's a duck.'

The medical resistance movement is led by the endocrinologists, who regard themselves as the high priests of modern, lab-centered medicine. As will be explained later, they overlook the crucial principle of testosterone resistance in the body. This is strange as many of these specialists also treat patients with diabetes, which in the majority of cases, as has been established for over seventy years, is due to resistance to the hormone insulin. If this key cause of diabetes had not been accepted by doctors fifty years ago before insulin could be measured but instead had been found to be high, according to the same logic, the hormone would have been denied to many patients to this day with disastrous consequences.

More evidence for testosterone resistance being the key to diagnosis and treatment will be given later. The fact remains that of the 20 percent of men over the age of fifty with symptoms of testosterone deficiency, only 1 percent are getting testosterone treatment in the UK and even less throughout Europe.[2] If this were thyroid-hormone deficiency and treatment rates, there would be a national and international outcry. But because of what I call testosterone resistance among medical professionals, deficiency of this hormone goes unrecognized and untreated, like the proverbial elephant in the doctor's consulting room. Let's see why this is and how we can do better.

Time Line of Testosterone Replacement Treatment (TRT)

Just over seventy-five years ago, within four months of one another, three groups from Holland, Germany, and Switzerland succeeded between them in isolating, characterizing, and then synthesizing the male hormone, testosterone. Within a couple of years, around about the time I was born, it began to be used clinically to relieve the characteristic symptoms of the male climacteric, or andropause, and other medical conditions such as heart and circulatory diseases and diabetes as well.

I would like to give you a sense of the ups and downs of testosterone treatment in my lifetime and why it may finally be accepted for its important role in both preventive medicine and treatment.

In the first few years, testosterone treatment was available as short-acting injections, which had to be given three times a week, or as long-acting pellet implants of fused crystals of testosterone and, unfortunately, as an oral preparation—toxic to the liver—called methyltestosterone, only taken off the market ten years ago in the USA. Even with this limited range of preparations, testosterone treatment became quite popular in the States in the 1940s but never really caught on in the UK. What could possibly go wrong?

World War II gave us other things to think about than treatment with hormone preparations manufactured in Germany, and postwar, it was back to basic medicine. When I qualified in 1960 and went into general practice, there was only oral methyltestosterone available for men with reduced libido, and the NHS didn't encourage prescription of that. About that time, medicine became overly 'scientific', with everyone busy measuring things in blood, and in fact, if you couldn't measure *it*, it didn't exist or was psychological. At that time, I left the bedside for the laboratory bench to train as a chemical pathologist.

Though I ended up working as a consultant in the department of steroid endocrinology at St Mary's Hospital in Paddington, I did my MD degree on stress, tension, and heart disease, measuring adrenaline (epinephrine) and noradrenaline (norepinephrine) together with fats, such as cholesterol, neutral fat, and free fatty acids, in the blood of people in a wide variety of stressful situations.

We will see later how many of these stress-related factors play an important part in causing testosterone resistance. I have published this theory in *The Lancet* in 1969 under the title of 'Aggression and Atheroma'[3] and in the book *The Western Way of Death: Stress, Tension and Heart Disease* in 1974.[4] The message was, 'Wroth, reinforced by sloth and gluttony, is the major cause of heart disease' (figure1).

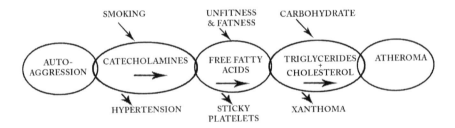

Figure 1. The chain of events linking stress to heart disease

Then in 1977, testosterone crossed my medical horizon in the form of a Danish doctor, Jens Møller, who against considerable opposition from his medical colleagues in Copenhagen University, who were loudly declaring such treatment to be 'hormonal humbug', was giving high-dosage testosterone injections to patients with serious circulatory problems in the legs.

What seriously annoyed his colleagues was that when they had done all the extensive arterial plumbing they could, and the toes and even whole limbs were going gangrenous and were ripe for amputation, the patients would go to Dr Møller's private clinic in the center of Copenhagen and get testosterone injections. This converted the limbs from painful, cold blue extremities to pink, painless, and fit for walking, while even skin ulcers and gangrene healed within a few weeks or months. This was inexplicable, in scientific medical terms, because it couldn't be recanalizing furred-up arteries, could it?

Recently, it has been shown that testosterone opens up the smaller collateral blood vessels to bypass the obstruction as well as causes favorable changes in metabolism, especially in diabetics.

I revisited his clinic in Copenhagen several times, and there was no denying the spectacular results he was getting with testosterone injections in saving limbs. You didn't need double-blind, placebo-controlled trials to assess the results. If you did a toe count and it remained stable for months and even years after the surgeons had decided that amputation was the only course of treatment, you were witnessing a major effect.

This experience encouraged me to leave the laboratory bench and return to the bedside in private practice about thirty years ago. Rather than having circulatory problems, the patients who came to see me had symptoms of testosterone deficiency best described as male menopause, or andropause, exactly as described by American doctors at the beginning of the 1940s.

Testosterone treatment by pills, pellets, or skin gels promptly relieved the characteristic symptoms of loss of energy, drive, and libido, depression, irritability, night sweats, and joint pains. This was most gratifying for doctors and patients alike.

Medical colleagues in general, especially endocrinologists, were much more antagonistic, and I encountered many skeptical and derisory comments at national and international meetings on testosterone. Also, for many years, I had silly debates on radio, television, and in the press on whether there was male menopause and if this 'monkey gland' treatment was just an expensive placebo sold to men looking for rejuvenation.

This was especially as the testosterone levels were often within the so-called laboratory normal range before treatment. Only later could I show that the laboratory ranges were variable and inaccurate, and the condition, like diabetes, could in the majority of cases be due to resistance to testosterone rather than an absolute lack of it.[5] This is a game changer as it justifies going much more on symptoms and their relief rather than arbitrary laboratory normal ranges. This theory is only gradually gaining acceptance and probably needs another five to ten years persistent pressure before it is accepted.

Though testosterone treatment has increased tenfold in the USA in the last year, it has flatlined in the UK and Australia under heavily biased legislation in the name of economy and hardline medical opinion (figure 2).

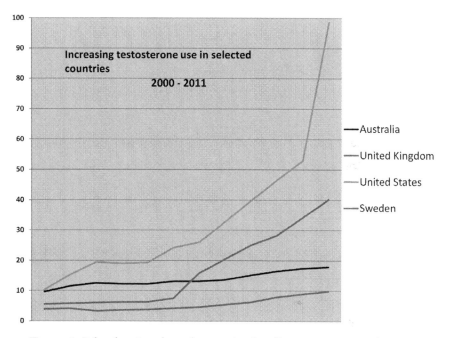

Figure 2. Sales data in selected countries for all testosterone products in defined doses per 1000 male population, showing fl at-lining in Australia and United kingdom compared to marked rises in USA and Sweden. (Statistics according to David Handlesman, Medical Journal of Australia, 199/8, (2013) 548-551).

What is really causing testosterone treatment to be taken much more seriously and helping it to become part of mainstream medicine is the evidence published over the last ten years that it can help control diabetes, reduce obesity, control heart disease symptoms, treat osteoporosis and some immunological disorders, and even possibly benefit early Alzheimer's disease and Parkinsonism. Its effectiveness in such conditions makes it more difficult to ignore.

This is combined with the greater access of both the medical professionals and the general public to information on the Internet about the symptoms and effects of testosterone deficiency and related conditions. People are increasingly able to make up their own minds and are less dependent on the high priests of endocrinology, unless treatment is denied to them by coercive legislation based on unreliable lab data and disease denial.

Also, because of falling testosterone levels seen in many populations worldwide, symptoms of deficiency of this key hormone and conditions related to it are on the increase.

I hope to be able to continue to bring you the good news on the rise and rise of testosterone treatment and the successful conclusion of a lifetime of its use in medicine.

But it's only been available for seventy-five years, so it's in its early days yet—give it time.

References for Introduction

[1] M. Carruthers, P. J. Cathcart, and M. R. Feneley, 'Evolution of Testosterone Treatment Over 25 Years: Symptom Responses, Endocrine Profiles, and Cardiovascular Changes', *The Aging Male* (2015).

[2] M. Carruthers, 'Time for International Action on Treating Testosterone Deficiency Syndrome', *The Aging Male*, 12/1 (2009), 21–28.

[3] M. E. Carruthers, 'Aggression and Atheroma', *The Lancet*, 2/7631 (1969), 1,170–1,171.

[4] M. Carruthers, *The Western Way of Death: Stress, Tension and Heart Disease* (London and New York: Davis-Poynter and Pantheon Books, 1974).

[5] M. Carruthers, 'The Paradox Dividing Testosterone Deficiency Symptoms and Androgen Assays: A Closer Look at the Cellular and Molecular Mechanisms of Androgen Action', *The Journal of Sexual Medicine*, 5/4 (2008), 998–1,012.

Chapter 1
Come Back, Galileo, Medicine Needs You Now

You cannot teach a man anything; you can only help him find it within himself.

Galileo Galilei

Why Is Testosterone Deficiency Syndrome so Seldom Diagnosed or Treated?

As is usual, a *syndrome* in medicine can be defined as the association of several clinically recognizable features, including both signs and symptoms. It is derived from the Greek word συνδρομή (*sundromē*) and means 'concurrence of symptoms'.

Certainly, testosterone deficiency conforms to the definition of a syndrome because whatever its cause, whether sudden castration, antiandrogen drugs, or simply aging, the constellation of symptoms produced is highly characteristic, specific, and can usually be relieved by a therapeutic trial of testosterone replacement therapy (TRT). The typical identikit pattern of symptoms includes loss of energy, drive, and libido, erectile dysfunction, memory loss, irritability, and depression and is sometimes accompanied by night sweats and hot flushes.

The peak age of onset is around fifty. The similarity to the female menopause is striking and has resulted in it being called the male climacteric in the literature of the 1930s and '40s and the slightly derogatory term *male menopause* from the 1960s onwards. More recently, it has become known as andropause or, better still, testosterone deficiency syndrome because it is being recognized at a wider age range and in association with other diseases such as diabetes.

It's as if nature has decided to rapidly reduce the possibility of reproduction after age fifty by causing the marker of fertility in women to cease, the periods, and in men by reducing erectile power generally, decreasing morning erections in particular. When life expectancy was around fifty, which it was in Europe and America in the 1920s and '30s (and still is in men in some countries such as Russia and parts of Africa), then the symptoms in men over that age were regarded as normal aging.

Now that in many developed countries, healthy life expectancy, including a sexually active life for both sexes, has risen to over seventy and, in many, over eighty, the acceptable criteria of a good later life have changed.

Adding to this is the mounting evidence, particularly over the last ten years, that testosterone deficiency is associated with a host of serious physical diseases of later life, such as heart disease, obesity, diabetes, osteoporosis, and even Alzheimer's disease.

Faced with this evidence in an aging population, you may think that doctors will be eager to encourage treatment for men complaining of the typical symptoms of testosterone deficiency syndrome. Not a bit of it. They seem to be leaning over backward not to make this particular diagnosis. Only 1 percent of the 20 percent of men over the age of fifty who have moderate to severe symptoms of the condition are diagnosed or treated.[1] Many endocrinologists rate the frequency of the condition as only 2 percent of the male population in the forty-to-eighty-year-old age range.[2] If, as clinical experience and application of symptom questionnaires confirms, the figure is ten times greater, this is the most common hormonal disorder in men and yet the least frequently treated. Why does the orthodox medical establishment allow this to continue?

Firstly, they are entrenched in the dogma that to diagnose testosterone deficiency, there has to be a level of the hormone in the blood which is lower than the laboratory norm, together with symptoms.

This is regardless of the fact that all the studies using the standard questionnaire which covers these symptoms, the aging male symptom (AMS) questionnaire, shows that there is little or no relationship between symptoms and testosterone levels.[3] Therefore, you have to pick one or the other. Why insist on both when they are unrelated?

The usual reason given is that modern so-called scientific medicine prefers laboratory measurements rather than untidy things, like patient symptoms, regardless of the fact that it's the symptoms which make up the syndrome. Because the two don't correlate, clinicians say the symptom questionnaires are nonspecific. If you make the diagnosis from the symptomatic *syndrome* point of view, it's the lab tests which are nonspecific.

The lack of correlation between lab tests and the symptoms is due to several factors. The measurements made in the laboratory are largely invalid because the so-called normal ranges are variable between labs, countries, populations, and individuals.[4] Lab values for testosterone can fall by 15–30 percent after food.[5] It has recently been shown that Spanish men are archetypal 'high-T' guys so that like racing cars, they only feel and function well sexually on 'high-octane' hormonal fuel.

Lab results are also wrongly interpreted because they are log-normally distributed, but this technical point can drag a sufferer into the 'normal range' and deny him testosterone treatment. Those lab-centered physicians who base their dogma tent on the slippery slope of testosterone values are also faced with the uncomfortable fact that several studies have shown that *normal ranges* are decreasing decade by decade so that on average, men have one-third less testosterone in the blood than their fathers at the same age.[6]

Also, there is the key factor of testosterone resistance comparable to insulin resistance seen in adult-onset diabetics,[7] giving one of the reasons for the title of this book. This resistance to the production and action of testosterone is a new concept that has been overlooked by the medical profession in general because it makes it possible for a man to have normal or even high levels of testosterone but still be relatively deficient because of his needs at that time and have the corresponding symptoms accordingly.

The regulation of the production of testosterone and its action is a complex relation operating at many levels in the body, few of which can be routinely measured in clinical practice.[8] The pituitary feedback mechanism and a protein which binds the sex hormones increase with age to a variable extent and is affected by various dietary and drug-related factors. Testosterone receptors can vary in number and sensitivity between individuals and races and interact with the many complex factors which regulate the action of testosterone and its derivatives within the cell.

This is where Galileo would come in useful, changing the worldview of doctors from the simplistic, lab-centered dogma, where the diagnosis of testosterone deficiency is made by measuring the testosterone level in the blood, to the new, patient-centered view. It is made by assessing the patient's symptoms by a questionnaire such as the aging male symptom (AMS) scale and, if there is a moderate or high score on this, giving a therapeutic trial of testosterone treatment. If the identikit pattern of symptoms goes away and stays away, most patients will feel the right diagnosis has been made regardless of complex and expensive laboratory tests which often deny it.

This is reminiscent of Galileo's fight against orthodoxy to make the sun the center of the solar system, the heliocentric view, rather than an immobile earth. This is the patient-centered view, which needs to replace the lab-centered view. The difference can be pictured as follows:

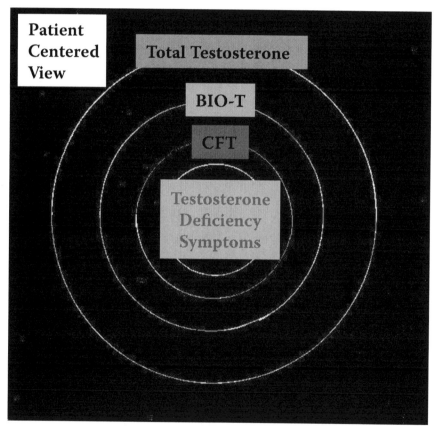

Figure 1. The patient-centered view of diagnosing testosterone deficiency (bioavailable testosterone (Bio-T), calculated free testosterone (CFT))

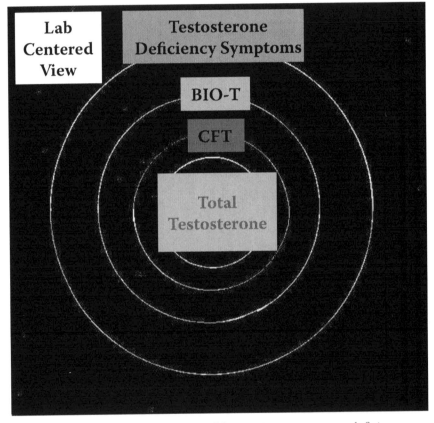

Figure 2. The lab-centered view of diagnosing testosterone deficiency

References for Chapter 1

[1] M. Carruthers, 'Time for International Action on Treating Testosterone Deficiency Syndrome', The Aging Male, 12/1 (2009), 21–28.

[2] I. Huhtaniemi, 'Late-Onset Hypogonadism: Current Concepts and Controversies of Pathogenesis, Diagnosis, and Treatment', Asian Journal of Andrology, 16/2 (2014), 192–202.

[3] M. Carruthers, P. J. Cathcart, and M. R. Feneley, 'Evolution of Testosterone Treatment Over 25 Years: Symptom Responses, Endocrine Profiles, and Cardiovascular Changes', The Aging Male (2015).

[4] M. Carruthers, T. R. Trinick, and M. J. Wheeler, 'The Validity of Androgen Assays', The Aging Male, 10/3 (2007), 165–172.

[5] M. Lehtihet, S. Arver, I. Bartuseviciene, and A. Pousette, 'S-Testosterone Decrease after a Mixed Meal in Healthy Men Independent of SHBG and Gonadotropin Levels', Andrologia (2012).

[6] A. M. Andersson, T. K. Jensen, A. Juul, J. H. Petersen, T. Jorgensen, and N. E. Skakkebaek, 'Secular Decline in Male Testosterone and Sex Hormone Binding Globulin Serum Levels in Danish Population Survey', Journal of Clinical Endocrinology and Metabolism, 92/12 (2007), 4,696–4,705.

[7] M. Carruthers, 'The Paradox Dividing Testosterone Deficiency Symptoms and Androgen Assays: A Closer Look at the Cellular and Molecular Mechanisms of Androgen Action', The Journal of Sexual Medicine, 5/4 (2008), 998–1,012.

[8] Ibid.

Chapter 2
Testosterone Treatment—
An Idea Whose Time Has Come ?

It is dangerous to be right when the government is wrong.

Voltaire

The experiences of patients seeking testosterone treatment in different countries vary widely according to the historic attitude of the doctors in that particular area.

Over sixty years after the hormone was first synthesized and used therapeutically, the year 2000, symbolically heralding the bright, new, forward-looking millennium, was a turning point in the history of testosterone treatment for several reasons. This was particularly because of the evidence of its effectiveness and safety presented at the Second World Congress on the Aging Male held in Geneva in February.

Also, in March there was a rare paper in the *British Medical Journal* which helped in turning the tide of medical opinion, favoring recognition of the andropause.[1] This was regarded as so important by American physicians that it was reprinted in its entirety as editor's choice in the *Western Journal of Medicine* in August 2000.[2]

The year ended with another important event, the launch conference of the Andropause Society (TAS) at the Royal Society of Medicine on 6 December. This was then a new, web-based international charity with the aims of encouraging research, education, and training about andropause and its treatment (www. andropause.org.uk). It has recently changed its name to Society for the Study of Androgen Deficiency to reflect the importance of these hormones related to testosterone in the causation and treatment of an ever-widening circle of diseases. These include diabetes, obesity, high blood pressure, circulatory diseases, and neurological conditions such as Alzheimer's disease and Parkinson's disease.

On the basis of a national survey of Canadian doctors and the confident assessment of the national and international scene by the society, the home page of the Canadian Andropause Society website starts with this encouraging statement:

> The existence of Andropause is now recognized by the medical world—including the Canadian Andropause Society—and by Canadians alike.

How had this victory in the worldwide testosterone revolution been won in Canada? As I saw when visiting the then president of the Canadian Andropause Society, Dr Tremblay, in Quebec in the autumn of 2000, he encouraged public awareness of the andropause and its treatment by press and television interviews. He also tirelessly traveled around Canada, as did Dr Alvaro Morales and several other members of his committee, attending and speaking at meetings of andrologists, endocrinologists, and general physicians. This high level of activity in making the case for treatment of the andropause inside and outside the medical profession bore the fruits of an increased level of acceptance in both.

Combined with an ongoing research and teaching program, this made the Canadian Andropause Society a model for organizations with similar goals around the world.[3] Unfortunately, it also caused an increase in the cheap and effective but toxic oral form of methyltestosterone. Though it has since been taken off the market in most countries around the world, it still was the commonest form of treatment in Canada, as found in a survey conducted in 2014[4], accounting for 36 percent of prescriptions.

Then in 2015, the wheel of public opinion went full circle. This time, under the banner of the Canadian Men's Health Foundation's Prof Alvaro Morales, a very experienced physician in the field who chaired the group. There was cautious recommendation of TRT for the treatment of the typical symptoms of testosterone deficiency which can wreck the family and working lives of many men. They emphasized that it might take one to two years of carefully monitored treatment for full symptom remission.

Even this modest suggestion from established leader in the field immediately drew a hostile flurry of ill-informed and intentioned press comments, trying to set the clock back twenty-five years. These ranged from the belittling question of 'Is there a male menopause?' and accusations that pharma-funded courses on TRT downplay risks and lead to overprescription in older men. These accusations are put in sensationalized terms as being 'part of a wave of courses touting the dubious virtues of testosterone treatment—all bankrolled by companies that manufacture the products'.

Worst still, according to these reports, many of the physicians taking time off from their busy practices to perjure their immortal souls do so for modest fees regardless of the fact that like priests, they should be doing it all for love. What other group in the society of highly respected professionals will be expected to do so while coming under such criticism for saying what they obviously sincerely believe?

Europe

Though a large amount of excellent research has been done in Europe over the last fifteen years, particularly in Scandinavia, in Italy, and to some extent, in the UK, as far as the actual application of testosterone is concerned, this is a backward area. Not only are GPs in the UK not allowed to start testosterone treatment, they also have to refer the patient to a hospital consultant who routinely rejects the request on the basis not of symptoms but of arbitrary lab results. The deciding factor of the local lower limit of total testosterone can go down to 4.3 nmol/L, according to one NHS lab in the Midlands.

This fallacious approach to diagnosis was given the seal of approval by a huge and expensive study of over 3,000 men aged forty to seventy-nine conducted at eight centers in Europe, the European Male Aging Study (EMAS), designed to establish once and for all official ranges for *normal* testosterone values and their relationship to the lifestyle of the participants.[5]

The conclusions were that the normal range, without the log correction patently needed, had a lower limit of 8 to 11 nmol/L, which gave a testosterone deficiency incidence of 2–5 percent, depending how many sexual symptoms you included in the diagnosis. Compared to the over 20 percent of cases you would expect in men over fifty according to prevalence of the characteristic symptoms, this lab-based approach is obviously missing a large number of men who could benefit from TRT.

Russia

In Russia, a brilliant young woman professor of endocrinology called Svetlana Kalinchenko, in 2004, realized that Russia was lagging behind many other countries in the use of testosterone, and invited me and my colleagues in the Andropause Society to give a training course in testosterone treatment. This course, which was held in Moscow in the early winter that year, was a great success and established me, as Svetlana jokingly said, as being 'the father of testosterone treatment in Russia'. She also got *The Testosterone Revolution* book published in Russian.

Though the welcome was very warm and the hospitality great, if the aim were to make the treatment available to men at all levels of the society, it was a failure. This was because the cheapest form of testosterone treatment, all that the average man could afford, was oral tablets of methyltestosterone. This was, as we emphasized in the lectures on the course, toxic to the liver, causing inflammation and jaundice as well as being harmful to the heart.

The nearly a hundred doctors from all over Russia on the course took this message to heart and stopped prescribing methyltestosterone and, where patients could afford it, used the much-safer long-acting injections of testosterone undecanoate (Nebido).

Unfortunately, as we found out three years later on follow-up courses in Moscow and Saint Petersburg, this stopped the poorer men in the population from getting the cheap oral preparation but increased the uptake of safer forms of testosterone treatment by the relatively rich. This switchover is shown in the graph of the number of packs of various preparations sold in Russia from 2001 to 2007 so that overall, the total number of preparations dispensed decreased, which was not the result we hoped for (figure 1). Still, with the advent of cheaper transdermal preparations, the long-term outlook for TRT in Russia may be better.

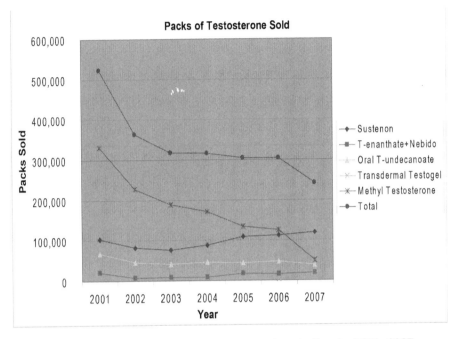

Figure 1. Sales of all testosterone preparations in Russia, 2001–2007

Asia and the Pacific Area

From the very limited knowledge and activity before the year 2000, this whole area has become a hive of interest in the health of the older man and the potential for male HRT. As was made clear at the historic First Asian Meeting of the International Society for the Study of the Aging Male, held in Kuala Lumpur, Malaysia, in March 2001, this focused very much on 'managing aging populations—a global challenge'.

Typical of the many excellent papers from delegates from every country in the region was a message from the organizing chairman, Dr H. M. Tan:[6]

In the developed countries, the percentage of the population of around 65 years of age will increase by more than 50% by the year 2025. The greatest rate of increase will be for the age group of above 80 years. With declining unsustainable birth rates, the traditional working population (age group 18–65 years) will face a huge burden if they have to fully support this aged population. Similarly, developing countries like China and Indonesia will experience the highest increase in the number of people above the age of 65 years. Their aged populations will more than double in size in the next 25 years. The sheer immensity of numbers will certainly strain the developing economies and their related social and political infrastructures.

Thus the problem of the aging population is universal, and in Asia where the majority of the countries are in the developing status, these problems may well be insurmountable if policy makers do not implement urgent and drastic steps well before this phenomenon occurs.

This sense of urgency was also conveyed by other speakers from every part of Asia, and one got the sense that each was ready and eager for what I called the testosterone revolution to happen in their country.

Indonesia was facing the most severe problem with a forecast increase of over 414 percent in its aged population in the years 2000–2025. Next came Kenya with 347 percent; Brazil, 255 percent; China, 220 percent; Japan, 129 percent, compared to the relatively modest increases in developed countries such as Germany with

66 percent and Sweden, 33 percent. The contrast was stark, and the thirst for knowledge on how to apply male HRT to maintain physical and mental activity, health span rather than just life span, was great.

While the knowledge of the nine invited speakers from the West was much sought and appreciated, there appeared to be less concern about the theory of testosterone treatment than the urgent need to apply it. Generally, while there was stronger support from the health authorities than was seen in most Western countries, who generally lack this sense of urgency, it fell to urologists to provide this form of HRT. The guidelines the Asian doctors recommended, however, closely followed the diagnostic and treatment criteria developed in the West. As indicated in the introduction, it is the pressure of aging populations which is creating the change in the climate of medical opinion needed to produce greater awareness of androgen deficiency and its treatment.

Australia

Despite the macho *"Crocodile" Dundee* image of the Australian male, Australia is as starved of testosterone treatment as it is of water.

Legislation was introduced via the Pharmaceutical Benefits Scheme (PBS) to prevent anyone but hospital specialists from prescribing TRT. Worse still, from 1 April 2015, it could only be given under a threshold of 6 nmol/L (167 ng/dL), half that allowed in most European countries.

It was also guaranteed to prevent 98 percent of the men suffering symptoms of testosterone deficiency from getting the treatment. This therapeutic nihilism extended to creating a climate of fear in doctors wishing to prescribe testosterone for symptoms of testosterone deficiency by arranging tribunal hearings of doctors prescribing outside the guidelines, which could result in a halt to their previous safe and effective practice of TRT, to the distress of many of their patients.

This is especially surprising as much of the research coming out of the leading andrology unit in Sydney appears to support the importance of maintaining a healthy blood testosterone level. In the summaries of work coming out of this one laboratory over the last ten years we read the following seemingly conflicting quotes:

1. 'Our findings show that decline in androgen status is associated with cognitive decline in older men.'[7]

2. 'E2 (derived from testosterone) is inversely associated with bone turnover markers—and bone remodeling is an independent marker of reduced diabetes risk.'[8]

3. 'Optimal androgen levels are a biomarker for survival.'[9]

4. 'Low serum T and E1 are associated with poorer self-rated health in older men.'[10]

5. 'Circulating androgens are more related to age and metabolic factors than CVD or chronic disease.'[11]

6. 'Higher plasma T or DHT is a biomarker for reduced risk of stroke but not myocardial infarction. Androgen exposure may influence outcomes after rather than the incidence of MI, whereas androgens but not E2 are independent predictors of stroke risk.'[12]

7. 'Men with a family history of T2DM were more susceptible to deleterious outcomes of overfeeding with greater reductions in serum testosterone and DHT and

greater increases in markers of insulin resistance, which may contribute to increased risk of developing type 2 diabetes.'[13]

8. 'Lowered circulating androgens (T and DHT) may be biomarkers rather than causally related to incident metabolic syndrome.'[14]

9. 'Low T, E2, and E1 were significantly associated with prospective functional decline over 2 years.'[15]

10. 'Aromatization plays only a minimal role in maintenance of sexual function in healthy eugonadal middle-aged or older men, but age and obesity (related to T) are significantly associated with decreases in most aspects of self-reported sexual function and satisfaction.'[16]

In spite of evidence coming from that one laboratory alone, a recent editorial in *Medical Care* describes any enthusiasm for TRT as a 'bubble about to burst'. To give it credence, it is accompanied by an article looking at prescribing in the veterans administration at Boston University, which airs the usual establishment concerns on unwarranted prescribing and their demands for diagnosis and treatment to be according to testosterone levels which we have shown to be invalid. All this is done in the name of public health advocacy and demands 'regular refreshment of strategic action' to check 'unjustified prescribing'.

With what, in the face of the evidence in favor of TRT, can only be described as a 'hormonophobic' attitude, this article states, 'A major step forward to reinforce the FDA's laudable initiatives in tightening restrictions on testosterone prescribing would be for professional societies to resume their neglected responsibilities and restore proper definition of "hypogonadism" that clearly distinguishes between pathologic and functional causes of low circulating testosterone.'

This approach to TRT is best summed up in a recent article called 'Mechanisms of Action of Testosterone—Unraveling a Gordian Knot.'[17] This reference is often used for an intractable problem easily solved by thinking outside the box, thus cutting the Gordian knot as Alexander did with his sword.

In this case, the puzzle of testosterone action in the clinical setting cannot be unraveled by clever, intellectual argument dreamed up by endocrinologists but simply needs cutting by the sword of truth, in this case the concept of testosterone resistance.

References for Chapter 2

[1] D. C. Gould, R. Petty, and H. S. Jacobs, 'For and Against: The Male Menopause—Does It Exist?', British Medical Journal, 320/7,238 (2000), 858–861.

[2] D. C. Gould, R. Petty, and H. S. Jacobs, 'The Male Menopause—Does It Exist?', Western Journal of Medicine, 173 (2000), 76–78.

[3] R. R. Tremblay and A. J. Morales, 'Canadian Practice Recommendations for Screening, Monitoring and Treating Men Affected by Andropause or Partial Androgen Deficiency', The Aging Male, 1/3 (1998), 213–218.

[4] S. A. Hall, G. Ranganathan, L. J. Tinsley, J. L. Lund, V. Kupelian, G. A. Wittert, et al., 'Population-Based Patterns of Prescription Androgen Use, 1976–2008', Pharmacoepidemiology and Drug Safety (2014).

[5] A. Tajar, I. T. Huhtaniemi, T. W. O'Neill, J. D. Finn, S. R. Pye, D. M. Lee, et al., 'Characteristics of Androgen Deficiency in Late-Onset Hypogonadism: Results from the European Male Aging Study (EMAS)', The Journal of Clinical Endocrinology and Metabolism, 97/5 (2012), 1,508–1,516.

[6] H. M. Tan, 'First Asian ISSAM Meeting: Managing Aging Populations—A Global Challenge', The Aging Male, 4, supplement 1 (2001), 7–12.

[7] B. Hsu, R. G. Cumming, L. M. Waite, F. M. Blyth, V. Naganathan, D. G. Le Couteur, et al., 'Longitudinal Relationships between Reproductive Hormones and Cognitive Decline in Older Men: The Concord Health and Ageing in Men Project', The Journal of Clinical Endocrinology and Metabolism, 100/6 (2015), 2,223–2,230.

8. B. B. Yeap, H. Alfonso, S. A. Chubb, R. Gauci, E. Byrnes, J. P. Beilby, et al., 'Higher Serum Undercarboxylated Osteocalcin and Other Bone Turnover Markers Are Associated with Reduced Diabetes Risk and Lower Estradiol Concentrations in Older Men', The Journal of Clinical Endocrinology and Metabolism, 100/1 (2015), 63–71.

9. B. B. Yeap, H. Alfonso, S. A. Paul Chubb, D. J., Handelsman, G. J. Hankey, O. P. Almeida, et al., 'In Older Men an Optimal Plasma Testosterone Is Associated with Reduced All-Cause Mortality and Higher Dihydrotestosterone with Reduced Ischemic Heart Disease Mortality, While Estradiol Levels Do Not Predict Mortality', The Journal of Clinical Endocrinology and Metabolism, 99/1 (2014), E9–E18.

10. B. Hsu, R. G. Cumming, F. M. Blyth, V. Naganathan, D. G. Le Couteur, M. J. Seibel, et al., 'Longitudinal and Cross-Sectional Relationships of Circulating Reproductive Hormone Levels to Self-Rated Health and Health-Related Quality of Life in Community-Dwelling Older Men', The Journal of Clinical Endocrinology and Metabolism, 99/5 (2014), 1,638–1,647.

11. B. B. Yeap, M. W. Knuiman, M. L. Divitini, D. J. Handelsman, J. P. Beilby, J. Beilin, et al., 'Differential Associations of Testosterone, Dihydrotestosterone and Oestradiol with Physical, Metabolic and Health-Related Factors in Community-Dwelling Men Aged 17–97 Years from the Busselton Health Survey', Clinical Endocrinology, 81/1 (2014), 100–108.

12. B. B. Yeap, H. Alfonso, S. A. Chubb, G. J. Hankey, D. J. Handelsman, J. Golledge, et al., 'In Older Men, Higher Plasma Testosterone or Dihydrotestosterone Is an Independent Predictor for Reduced Incidence of Stroke but Not Myocardial Infarction', The Journal of Clinical Endocrinology and Metabolism, 99/12 (2014), 4,565–4,573.

13. K. Sato, D. Samocha-Bonet, D. J. Handelsman, S. Fujita, G. A. Wittert, L. K. Heilbronn, 'Serum Sex Steroids and Steroidogenesis-Related Enzyme Expression in Skeletal Muscle During Experimental Weight Gain in Men', Diabetes and Metabolism, 40/6 (2014), 439–444.

14. B. Hsu, R. G. Cumming, V. Naganathan, F. M. Blyth, D. G. Le Couteur, M. J. Seibel, et al., 'Associations between Circulating Reproductive Hormones and SHBG and Prevalent and Incident Metabolic Syndrome in Community-Dwelling Older Men: The Concord Health and Ageing in Men Project', The Journal of Clinical Endocrinology and Metabolism, 99/12 (2014), E2686–E2691.

15. B. Hsu, R. G. Cumming, V. Naganathan, F. M. Blyth, D. G. Le Couteur, M. J. Seibel, et al., 'Longitudinal Relationships of Circulating Reproductive Hormone with Functional Disability, Muscle Mass, and Strength in Community-Dwelling Older Men: The Concord Health and Ageing in Men Project', The Journal of Clinical Endocrinology and Metabolism, 99/9 (2014), 3,310–3,318.

16. G. A. Sartorius, L. P. Ly, and D. J. Handelsman, 'Male Sexual Function Can Be Maintained without Aromatization: Randomized Placebo-Controlled Trial of Dihydrotestosterone (DHT) in Healthy, Older Men for 24 Months', The Journal of Sexual Medicine, 11/10 (2014), 2,562–2,570.

17. D. J. Handelsman, 'Mechanisms of Action of Testosterone—Unraveling a Gordian Knot', New England Journal of Medicine, 369/11 (2013), 1,058–1,059.

Chapter 3
Sources of Internal Resistance

"The fault, dear Brutus, is not in our stars,
But in ourselves, that we are underlings."

Shakespeare - Julius Caesar (I, ii, 140-141)

The fault causing this relative deficiency of testosterone is not in our testes as is commonly assumed, but in our cellular metabolism, especially the receptors, that are insensitive or resistant to the actions of the hormone.

This chapter is deliberately technical to give the full medical evidence for testosterone resistance. It can be skipped if the reader is willing to accept that there is plenty of scientific evidence about the existence of resistance to the multiple complex actions of testosterone in the body. It makes the point that there are many parallels between the accepted features of insulin resistance in diabetes and the controversial presence of testosterone resistance in adult-onset testosterone deficiency.

However there are many important figures to illustrate the text, and it is worth having a look at these as they explain the internal resistance concept concisely and represent the best in medical art in this field.

Introduction

In an elegant article entitled 'Mechanism of Diabetes Mellitus' published in *The Lancet* in 1939, Sir Harold Himsworth drew the distinction between insulin-sensitive and insulin-insensitive diabetes, shedding new light on the nature, diagnosis, and treatment of the condition.[1]

This chapter explores the possibility that similar principles may explain the different causes and endocrine background of what has become known as the testosterone deficiency syndrome (TDS). It also reviews the evidence that androgen resistance may be an important factor in the onset of this condition and may cause problems with its diagnosis and treatment.

Central Paradox in the Diagnosis of TDS

The typical symptoms of TDS have been recognized and consistent since they were first described nearly seventy years ago by Dr. August Werner (table 1).[2, 3, 4, 5, 6, 7]

The paradox is that these characteristic symptoms of testosterone deficiency are very poorly correlated with total testosterone (TT) or other androgen levels in the blood. A recent report on the best validated of all the symptom scales, the aging male symptoms (AMS) scale, states that 'the total AMS score was not significantly associated with TT.'[8] Similarly, using three questionnaires, including the AMS and androgen deficiency in the adult male, St Louis (ADAM) scales, no relationship was found between symptomatology and any of a battery of eight endocrine assays, including TT and free testosterone (FT), other than possibly age-related declines in dehydroepiandrosterone (DHEA) and insulin-like growth factor 1 (IGF-1).[9]

Further investigation of a group of eighty-one Belgian men aged fifty-three to sixty-six (mean fifty-nine) concluded 'there was no correlation between AMS (total and subscales) and testosterone levels,'[10] while the same group in a study of 161 more elderly men aged 74–89 (mean 78) also showed no correlation between symptom scores and TT, FT, or bioavailable testosterone (BT).[11]

However, possibly because the ADAM symptom scores may be more age-related than the AMS, in a study of men aged twenty-three to eighty years, unlike TT, BT and FT were found to correlate significantly with a number of the individual questions, both on that and the AMS scale.[12] Also, in an evaluation of assays measuring androgens over a similar wide age range, TT showed no correlation with age and, if taken alone, would have resulted in misclassification of deficiency in 42 percent when compared with BT.[13]

One of the studies most clearly highlighting the paradox dividing androgen deficiency symptom scales and laboratory measures is that of Miwa et al. in 2006, which found no correlation between the total and psychological, somatic, or sexual domain scores of the AMS and serum levels of TT, FT, estradiol (E2), luteinizing hormone (LH), follicle-stimulating hormone (FSH), dehydroepiandrosterone sulfate (DHEA-S), or growth hormone (GH).[14]

Similarly, while individual symptoms, such as reduced libido[15] or erectile dysfunction,[16] have some association with androgen levels in epidemiological studies, they do not appear to be related to them in individual cases,[17] and the different symptoms and metabolic effects appear at different levels—i.e., there seem to be various organ thresholds of sensitivity and, hence, possible pathology. Without any clear-cut threshold for overall symptoms of testosterone deficiency, there is a pattern of increasing prevalence of symptoms and metabolic risk factors with decreasing androgen levels.[18]

Author	Werner	Heller	Reiter	Carruthers	Carruthers	Tremblay	Heinemann
Year the study began	1938	1944	1963	UKAS 1989	Web 1996	1998	1999
Number in study	273	23	100	1,500	1,533	300	116
Reference number	[2]	[3]	[4]	[5]	[5]	[6]	[7]
Symptoms							
Erectile dysfunction	95	++	++	84	83	++	88
Libido / sex drive/ desire	90	++	++	82	87	++	84
Fatigue / energy reduced	76	++	+	76	94	+	80
Depression	89	+	++	60	88	+	75
Anxiety/ nervousness	100	++	++	++	85	+	69
Memory/ concentration	87	+	+	37	90	+	
Irritability/anger	59	+	+	54	85	+	72
Aches/pains joints	75	+		55	83		77
Sweating especially at night	35	+		49	63	+	66
Vasomotor/flushes	46	+		27		+	
Aging/older than years				40	55		59
Dry skin/thinning	30	+		39	63		

Table 1. Frequency of symptoms of testosterone deficiency syndrome described by various authors (2–7), where + = mentioned; ++ = frequent; UKAS = UK Androgen Study

In this study, androgen-induced prevalence of loss of libido or energy increased significantly below testosterone concentrations of 15 nmol/L (430 ng/dL), whereas depression and diabetes mellitus type 2 in non-obese men were more common with testosterone concentrations below 10 nmol/L (300 ng/dL). Erectile dysfunction was identified as a composite pathology of metabolic risk factors, smoking, and depressivity, whereas only testosterone concentrations below 8 nmol/L (230 ng/dL) contributed to that symptom.

The authors concluded that in this cohort from an andrology clinic, which might not be representative of the general population, symptoms accumulated gradually with decreasing testosterone levels and that various strata of TT concentrations exist, which are associated with specific symptoms.

Sexual responses to treatment, especially erectile function, have been found to vary according to initial TT and FT levels across a wide range of values, including in men with low-normal levels.[19] There is also a considerable variation between individuals in levels of testosterone at which symptoms appear. Kelleher et al.[20] investigated fifty-two androgen-deficient men who underwent 260 implantations over a five-year period. At the time of return of androgen deficiency symptoms, the blood TT and FT concentrations were highly reproducible within individuals, but each person had a consistent testosterone threshold for androgen deficiency symptoms that differed markedly between individuals.

Further divergence of symptoms and androgen levels is seen in population-screening studies and in the selection of androgen-deficient patients for trials of testosterone treatment. Symptom scales such as the AMS suggest an incidence of 40–50 percent in men over the age of fifty, but only between 1 and 7 percent of men with raised symptom scores prove to have testosterone levels sufficient to be declared hypogonadal and, therefore, suitable for treatment according to various international guidelines.

Despite this contradictory evidence, the lower limit of TT, which is regarded as diagnostic of androgen deficiency, varies between 6 nmol/L (176 ng/dL) in Australia[21] and 12 nmol/L (350 ng/dL) in Europe and the United States,[22, 23] with some trials accepting patients with levels up to 15 nmol/L (430 ng/dL) in an effort to recruit sufficient symptomatic subjects.

This review emphasizes the problems of diagnoses based on TT alone, especially considering the questionable validity of androgen assays overall when all the variables in sampling, analysis, and interpretation are taken into account.[24]

This dichotomy between clinical and laboratory findings urgently needs to be explained to reduce the confusion over what one does for men who have symptoms of androgen deficiency unsubstantiated by laboratory tests. For this, we need to take a detailed look at the multiple levels at which testosterone production and action can be impaired (figure 1).[25]

Levels at which Testosterone Resistance can occur
(Carruthers, M. J.Sex. Med., 5, 998-1012, 2008)

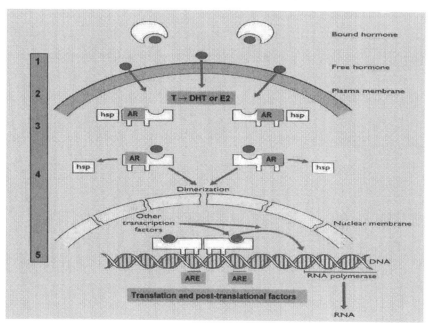

Figure 1. Impaired Androgen Synthesis and Regulation

Aging

The aging process affects androgen production and regulation at every level of the hypothalamo-gonadal axis (figure 2).[26] The reduction in TT and more, especially in both BT and CFT, with age is well recognized[27, 28, 29] and may be accelerating because of health and environmental effects.[30] As well as lower mean levels, there is a reduction in the circadian rhythm in older men.[31, 32]

Partly, this is because of a decrease in the efficacy of LH pulses in stimulating androgen production.[33] The question arises as to what proportion of these changes is due to testicular degeneration and how much to impaired regulation.

Testes: Impaired Development

Men with nondescent, or late descent, of one or both testes often show signs and symptoms of testosterone deficiency throughout their lives, and when testosterone treatment is stopped, they develop typical symptoms. Even when there has been anatomic correction of the defect by orchidopexy, testicular function may well still be impaired, both in terms of sperm and testosterone production.

Sometimes, there is no overt history of testicular problems, but when the patient presents in middle age or later, there may be a lifelong history of low sex drive and activity, unexplained infertility, and poor secondary sexual characteristics. Physical examination may show small easily retractile testes in a poorly developed scrotum, with a small penis.

Aging

A wide range of degenerative changes have been reported in the aging testis. These include a decrease in the number of Leydig cells, increased fibrosis, decreased perfusion, and hypoxia-dependent changes in steroidogenesis, resulting in reduced precursor DHEA synthesis (figure 2).[34, 35] As will be discussed later, testicular failure may also develop after a period of compensatory Leydig cell overactivity and hypertrophy.

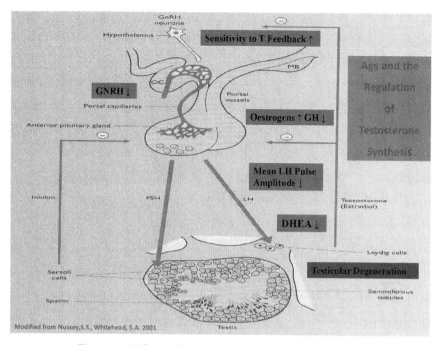

Figure 2. Effects of aging on testosterone production

Infections

Mumps is the classic example of an infection causing an endocrine disorder. Orchitis occurs in 25–35 percent of postpubertal cases and, like many testicular disorders, may affect its endocrine function as well as sperm production. This potential for testicular damage to be caused by a wide variety of viruses may be linked to damage to the immunological defense system of the testes, which is only established at puberty.

Other viruses, including those causing glandular fever (infectious mononucleosis), may also be associated with clinical or subclinical orchitis and damage. This has also been reported with herpes, coxsackievirus, arbovirus, and dengue and Marburg viruses. The testes can also be affected by nephritis, prostatitis, vesiculitis, and epididymitis, especially with gonorrhea, chlamydia, and other causes of nonspecific urethritis.

Temperature

Varicocele and hydroceles impair the temperature regulation function of the scrotum, which normally keeps the testes 3–4°C cooler than core body temperature, and about 1.5–2.5°C below the temperature of the scrotal skin.[36]

Many andrologists interested both in infertility and androgen deficiency encourage scrotal cooling measures such as the wearing of loose-fitting boxer shorts and avoidance of tight jeans[37] and prolonged periods of driving.[38]

Trauma

Testicular trauma as a cause of androgen deficiency is not always obvious from the history. It can include hernial repair at any age but particularly in infancy, when it may be an aspect of partial nondescent of the testes and impaired development of the inguinal canal. Direct blows to the testes, sufficient to cause bruising, may cause unilateral testicular atrophy, as can torsion, even when surgically corrected at an early stage. This may be due to either a breach in the immunological defenses of the testis or a prolonged sympathetic spasm that can affect both sides.

Similar mechanisms can account for testicular atrophy or hypofunction, which may follow any operation on the testis, particularly when it involves trauma to the capsule, as in removal of a varicocele or damage to the vas, particularly with vasectomy.[39] Operations on the prostate, including transurethral resection, may also damage the vas or their outflow, as shown by retrograde ejaculation of semen into the bladder, and may possibly cause an autoimmune orchitis.

Removal of one testis for testicular cancer, especially where there has been chemotherapy or radiation, or following herniorrhaphy may not be immediately followed by infertility or symptoms of testosterone deficiency.[40] However, these may appear later in life at a relatively early age because of a lower reserve of testicular function.

Heredity and Familial Influences

Studies of monozygotic and dizygotic twins[41] have shown that familial factors account for twice as much of the concordance in TT and FT and dihydrotestosterone (DHT) as genetic factors and virtually all sex hormone-binding globulin (SHBG) and aromatase activity. In all these factors, nurture appears more important than nature. Only in estradiol and luteinizing hormone levels does heredity have a slightly greater influence. It is suggested that similar diet and physical activity levels in families may explain most of these factors in determining androgen levels and, hence, liability to androgen deficiency.

Changes in the Regulation of Testosterone Synthesis

Advancing years take their toll on the brain as the biggest sex organ in the body in many ways. Psychologically, sexual stimuli tend to be less frequent and less intense. Feedback of sensory impulses from the wrinkled skin and flaccid penis creating arousal is similarly reduced. The reduced penile sensitivity has been shown to be due to lower testosterone levels and a reduction of the number of androgen receptors (ARs) in the penis.[42]

Physically, apart from neuronal dropout in the cortex and various brain nuclei mediating sexual activity, there can be an insidious cognitive impairment leading, in extreme case, to dementia. Lowered testosterone levels have been found in Alzheimer's disease,[43] stroke,[44] and Parkinson's disease.[45]

Stress

Both excessive and unpleasant physical and mental stress can suppress the hypothalamo-gonadal axis and can reduce either the production or activity of androgens.[46] For example, extreme endurance training in military cadets involving psychic stress and deprivation of food and sleep results in a marked drop in testosterone levels.[47]

Less-acute psychological stress, such as redundancy, divorce, financial problems, and loss of close friends or relatives, has been shown to lower androgen levels.[48] Retirement, boredom, bereavement, isolation, and illness also contribute to stress in the elderly.

Physical illnesses ranging from life-threatening trauma to a variety of chronic diseases have been found to reduce testosterone levels, although it is always difficult to establish which comes first.[49]

Alcohol

Although excess alcohol intake is well recognized as a cause of infertility, its short-term and long-term effects on testosterone production are often overlooked.

Long-term, in men, it has been found that moderate levels of stable alcohol intake (nonbinge drinking) has no adverse effects·

on gonadal function, as estimated by testosterone levels and the FT index.[50]

In contrast, excess alcohol intake, short- or long-term, has a variety of adverse effects on androgen status in men. Acutely, high doses cause a decrease in androgen levels by a variety of mechanisms. Partly, these are related to a direct inhibition of testosterone production by acetaldehyde derived from the metabolism of alcohol.[51] Also, alcohol suppresses luteinizing hormone-releasing hormone (LHRH) released by stimulating beta-endorphinergic neurons that inhibit the production of norepinephrine, which drives the nitric oxide-mediated release of LHRH.[52] However, majority of the endocrine effects of alcohol are probably indirect, resulting from either the stress of intoxication, with stimulation of cortisol, catecholamines, and prolactin, or changes in the level of intermediary metabolites, e.g. free fatty acids (FFA), resulting from alteration in intracellular redox state or tissue damage.[53]

Diet, Xenoestrogens, and Antiandrogens

Strict low-cholesterol diets have been shown to lower TT and FT levels by 14 percent.[54] Vegetarian diets, especially if low in protein, can increase SHBG, further reducing FT. However, men who put on a low-fat, high-fiber vegetarian diet have an 18 percent reduction in both TT and FT, which is reversed when they go back on a normal diet. This parallel reduction in both androgen measures seems to indicate that in this situation, the decrease is primarily in testosterone.[55] Conversely, high-protein, low-carbohydrate diets, such as the fashionable weight-reduction Atkins diet, and Dr Michael Mosley's new 'Fast Diet' may partly exert their slimming action by raising TT and lowering SHBG.

Drugs/Medications

As well as psychotropic drugs that interfere with gonadotropin-releasing hormone (GnRH) and LH production, there are many drugs that can directly reduce the production of androgens at the testicular level or can alter their metabolism.

Severe hyperprolactinemia, with consequent reductions in TT, sexual desire, and erectile function, has been found to be related to the use of antidepressants, antipsychotic drugs, and benzamides.[56]

Drugs such as aminoglutethimide and ketoconazole can inhibit steroidogenic enzymes, causing rapid and dramatic reductions in testosterone levels.[57]

Long-term use of phosphodiesterase type 5 (PDE5) inhibitors, such as tadalafil, has been found to increase the TT–E2 ratio, mainly by reducing E levels, considered because of 'androgen–estrogen cross-talk and possible inhibition of aromatase activity'.[58]

Oral hypoglycemic agents, especially the most frequently used glitazones, rosiglitazones (Avandia, GlaxoSmithKline, Research Triangle Park, New Hampshire, USA), and pioglitazones (Actos, Takeda, Osaka, Japan), by their action as peroxisome peroxidase gamma agonists, both reduce testosterone synthesis and raise SHBG, which together greatly decrease FT.[59, 60] While these actions can be beneficial in treating polycystic ovarian syndrome, in diabetics with already reduced testosterone levels, it may explain many of the adverse side effects of these drugs, especially on the heart,[61] and in causing anemia and osteoporosis.

Recently the adverse effects of drugs blocking the conversion of testosterone to dihydrotesterone by 5α reductase inhibition, as used in various hair restoring products, have come into prominence as a cause of long-lasting loss of libido and erectile dysfunction in young men, a so-called post-finasteride syndrome.

Level 2—Androgen Binding to Plasma Proteins

Of the TT circulating in the blood, 40–50 percent is weakly bound to albumin, and 50–60 percent is strongly bound to SHBG. Only 1–3 percent of the hormone is free (FT) and, together with the albumin-bound fraction, is referred to as the BT.

The albumin-bound fraction of testosterone and its metabolites estradiol (E2) and DHT are thought to be biologically available to all tissues and organs. However, the availability of this fraction of the hormones varies widely among different organs according to the capillary transit time in relation to the dissociation constants of the binding proteins and the rate of diffusion through the capillary wall.[62, 63]

SHBG regulates not only the absolute but also the relative amounts of sex steroids available to tissues because it is an 'estradiol amplifier',[64] having a fivefold greater affinity for testosterone. This explains why with age, as SHBG levels rise in men, FT levels fall, and as evidence of greater estrogenic action, both benign enlargement of the prostate and gynecomastia become more common conditions. Also, estrogenic feedback on the pituitary-gonadal axis inhibits testosterone production by the testes (figure 2).

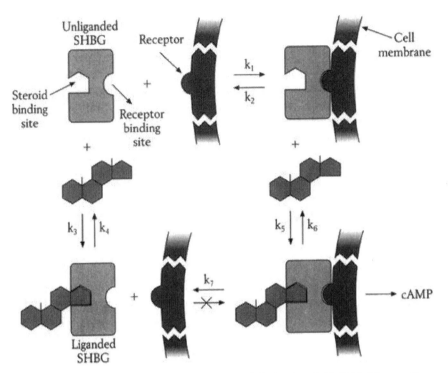

Figure 3. The steroid sex hormone binding globulin (SHBG)-SHBGR signaling system

Regulation of SHBG Protein Expression

Given the pivotal role of SHBG in regulating the activity of the sex steroids by sequestering them in the bound state, it is important to recognize the factors that modulate SHBG levels (table 2).

Table 2. Summary of Factors Influencing Sex Hormone-Binding Globulin Synthesis and Sex Steroid Binding

Increased by
- Age
- Estrogens and xenoestrogens
- Glucocorticoids

- Thyroxine

- Free fatty acids (FFAs), especially saturated FFA

- Drugs, e.g. anticonvulsants

Decreased by
- Androgens

- Insulin and obesity

- Growth hormone

- Diet—high protein and low carbohydrate

- Drugs, e.g. Danazol

Cellular Actions of SHBG

In addition to its function as a steroid-binding protein and estrogen amplifier, SHBG also functions as part of a novel steroid-signaling system that is independent of the classical intracellular steroid receptors. Recent research has shown that SHBG is a modular protein which comprises an N-terminal steroid-binding and dimerization domain and a C-terminal domain containing a highly conserved consensus sequence for glycosylation that may be required for other biological activities such as cell-surface recognition.[65]

Unlike the intracellular steroid receptors that are hormone-activated transcription factors, SHBG mediates androgen and estrogen, signaling at the cell membrane via a cyclic adenosine monophosphate-dependent (cAMP-dependent) pathway (figure 3).[66] That this is a separate pathway of steroid action is shown by the fact that inhibitors of the transcriptional activation of the AR and estrogen receptor do not affect the cAMP response.[67]

In the prostate, it has been suggested that the estradiol-activated SHBG / sex hormone-binding globulin receptor (SHBG-R) complex cross-talks with the AR and is able to activate the AR even in the absence of DHT.[68] These factors may be of importance in relation to the actions of androgens and estrogens in the causation and treatment of both benign and malignant prostatic disorders.

Level 3—Reduced Tissue Responsiveness

Structural Changes

Aging produces changes in many tissues which reduce their responses to androgenic stimulation. Most of the research in this area has been focused on the structural changes in the penis with age and androgen deprivation, for obvious clinical and commercial reasons.

Testosterone stands at the crossroads in the evolution of stromal precursor cells, directing their differentiation toward muscle tissue, whether smooth or striated, rather than the default state of adipose tissue (figure 4). Therefore, androgens exert a direct effect on penile tissue to maintain erectile function, and deficiency produces metabolic and structural imbalances in the corpus cavernosum, resulting in venous leakage and erectile dysfunction.[69]

Actions of Testosterone on Cell Differentiation and Activity

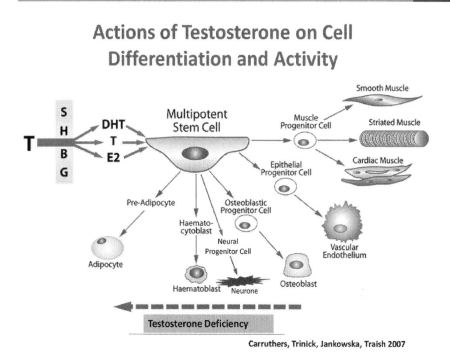

Carruthers, Trinick, Jankowska, Traish 2007

Figure 4. Action of testosterone on the differentiation of multipotent stem cells

Fortunately, as with the reduction in muscle mass and accumulation of visceral fat seen in diabetes and metabolic syndrome, these changes are reversible by androgen treatment, with a consequent improvement in erectile function.[70, 71, 72, 73]

Decreased blood flow to many tissues with age also reduces the supply of testosterone to the cells.[74] Endothelial damage as part of the accelerated atherosclerosis seen in androgen-deficient states has been shown to be associated with a decrease in arterial inflow to the penis[75] and is reversed by testosterone treatment.

The number of ARs in various tissues has been shown to decrease with age, and these can also undergo downregulation.[76] There are neurovascular changes, particularly in diabetics, which further reduce tissue responsiveness.

Tissue-Specific Prereceptor Actions

When testosterone enters the cell, variable amounts are converted to the metabolically more active form, DHT, by 5α-reductase enzymes and to estrogen by aromatase enzymes. With age and because of the action of 5α-reductase inhibitors such as dutasteride and finasteride, DHT levels both in the circulation and in the cells can be decreased. Conversely, with age and obesity, aromatase levels can be increased, causing suppression of testosterone production via the hypothalamo-gonadal axis and antagonizing its action in the cells.

Within the cells, androgens also regulate the complex enzymatic machinery in endothelial and smooth muscle cells, which affects both the structure and function of their cytoskeleton (figure 4). In the penis, for example, the RhoA/Rho kinase pathway, a mediator of cavernosal smooth muscle contraction, is inhibited by androgens, which stimulate the action of nitric oxide synthase (figure 5).[77] This at least partly explains the synergistic action of testosterone and PDE5 inhibitors[78, 79, 80] and why in diabetes, where of the two isoforms of Rho kinase, only type 1 is increased in penile tissue, androgen treatment is effective in normalizing this pathway and restoring erectile function.[81]

CAG (poly-glutamine) Variations

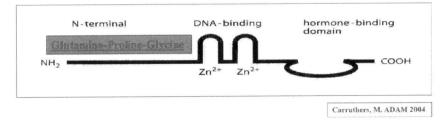

Figure 5. The much mutated androgen receptor

Metabolic Changes

Androgen deficiency has been shown to decrease lipid oxidation and resting energy expenditure, raising FFA, triglycerides, and cholesterol and increasing insulin resistance.[82] These data indicate that low serum testosterone levels are associated with an adverse metabolic profile, erectile dysfunction, and increased cardiovascular risk[83, 84] and suggest a novel unifying mechanism for the previously independent observations that androgen deficiency and impaired mitochondrial function promote insulin resistance in men.

Level 4—AR Activity

Genetic mutations in the AR have been shown to affect genital development, prostate tissue, spermatogenesis, bone density, hair growth, cardiovascular risk factors, psychological factors, insulin sensitivity, TT, SHBG, and FT levels.

CAG-repeat lengths vary normally between eighteen and twenty-four—the greater the length, the more the androgen resistance, and in extreme cases, complete androgen insensitivity can cause complete loss of male phenotype in the androgen insensitivity syndrome. Longer mutations can also arise in prostate cancer, especially when it is metastatic or has become hormone resistant (figure 5).[85]

Asian races, with twenty-two to twenty-three CAG repeats, have lower TT, SHBG, and FT with greater insulin resistance, more diabetes, and less prostate cancer than Afro-Caribbeans, with eighteen to twenty repeats, higher TT, SHBG, and FT, and half the insulin resistance but more prostate cancer. White Europeans with twenty-one to twenty-two are intermediate in all these factors.

Strong positive correlations have been found between CAG-repeat lengths, TT, FT, and LH and are attributed to differences in androgen sensitivity and feedback set point.[86]

GGN (Polyglycine) Variations

It has been shown both in vivo and in vitro that small differences in the length of the GGN codon can have marked effects on the activity of the AR, particularly when combined with longer CAG-repeat lengths.

A study of infertile men in Sweden has shown that those with twenty-four GGN repeats have lower testicular volumes and decreased seminal prostate-specific antigen (PSA) and zinc compared to those with twenty-three repeats, and concludes that the former is associated with relative androgen resistance.[87]

The same Scandinavian group has also found that unlike normal men, boys with hypospadias more often have AR gene with twenty-four rather than twenty-three repeats.[88] Longer GGN-repeat lengths can also be linked to androgen resistance and may be the cause of TDS, which includes testicular maldescent, hypospadias, testicular cancer, and infertility. This is sometimes summarized as 'a bad testis' and attributed to the greater sensitivity of this genome to adverse environmental influences ranging from maternal smoking to organochloride pollutants.

It has been shown in vitro that ARs with other glutamine numbers than twenty-three have lower transactivating capacity in response to both testosterone and DHT, and it is suggested that these can be linked to congenital malformations and other signs of a lower AR activity.[89]

In these ways, minor variations in the AR gene can have major consequences in deciding the structure and function of androgen-responsive tissues throughout life. Referring to the variations in the CAG repeats, Zitzmann and Nieschlag state that 'this modulation of androgen effects may be small but continuously present during a man's lifetime and, hence, exerts effects that are measurable in many tissues as various degrees of androgenicity and represents a relevant effector of maleness'.[90] With the inclusion of variations in glycine residues, this leads to a theory of the overall genetic regulation of androgen action within a particular individual.

Other Factors Affecting the AR

While the number of ARs increases with puberty, with age there is a decrease, especially in genital tissue. Upregulation and downregulation of ARs are known to occur with sustained decreases and elevations of androgen levels. A wide variety of xenoestrogens and antiandrogens is known to occur especially in agrochemicals, and antiandrogenic drugs are used in the treatment of prostate cancer.

There are two zinc fingers on the binding domain of each AR, and clinical zinc deficiency may impair binding. Zinc is also reported to inhibit the activity of the aromatase enzymes in the cell, limiting the conversion of testosterone to estrogen.[91]

Level 5—Transcription and Translation Factors

Over fifty different transcription factors are known to bind to the promoter/enhancer or repressor sites for the steroid hormone receptors and affect their ability to activate RNA polymerase. The stability and availability of these proteins are largely regulated by heat shock proteins (HSP) grouped into families according to their molecular size.

Hsp as ARs

Hsp90 is required for the maintenance of an active conformation in hormone-bound AR to regulate nuclear transfer, nuclear matrix binding, and transcriptional activity.

Pure antiandrogens block the transconformational change of AR in an intermediary complex, unable to acquire the active conformation and to dissociate the Hsp90.

Proteins that interact with both Hsp90 and Hsp70 families lead to a large decrease in AR activity by slowing their rate of synthesis and reducing their rate of breakdown.[92]

Coactivators and Corepressors

AR function is specifically modulated by transcriptional coregulators or corepressors that interact with a host of other transcription factors to either activate or repress the transcription of specific genes. These coactivators/corepressors act by modifying the chromatin structure/function and making the associated DNA either more or less accessible to RNA polymerase transcription. One major class of transcription coregulators modifies the chromatin structure through covalent modification of histones, the histone acyltransferases. A second, adenosine triphosphate-dependent (ATP-dependent) class remodels the chromatin structure.

The complex functions of many coregulators of transcription are under intensive investigation because of their possible role in a wide range of disease processes, including both male and female reproductive aging, and associated pathophysiological processes, such as prostate cancer.[93]

Posttranslational Factors

At the final step of androgen action after transcription by RNA polymerase, within the DNA spiral, histone-regulated acetylation, ubitylation, and sumoylation all play important roles in modulating AR function. The acetylation of the AR is induced by dihydrotestosterone and by histone deacetylase inhibitors.[94]

Conclusions

Etiology of TDS

The many parallels and interactions between maturity-onset diabetes and TDS suggest that a combination of lack of testosterone and its metabolites, combined with resistance to its action at multiple levels, underlies the pathology of androgen deficiency. Just as insulin resistance is thought to vary between tissues, so is androgen resistance, and therefore, different organs may respond functionally or metabolically with differing consequences.

As in diabetes, there can be genetic predispositions to androgen deficiency, both racial and familial, which interacts with lifestyle and disease-related factors. Similarly, after a period of compensation, the ability of the testis to overcome the androgen resistance may fail, with structural changes in the Leydig cells and signs and symptoms of endocrine failure developing.

In particular, there is a similarity between the changes observed in the testis with aging and with the pancreatic islets in maturity-onset diabetes. Type 2 diabetes is associated with raised and then lowered insulin levels combined with insulin resistance. This is due to the failure of beta cell compensatory hypertrophy or hyperplasia. Prolonged stimulation of the beta cells depletes the insulin granule stores and causes amyloid deposition in the islets (glucotoxicity). Beta cells become unable to secrete pulses of insulin and are then 'blind' to changes in glucose concentration. Hyperglycemia also contributes to insulin resistance as a result of downregulation, with decreased numbers of glucose transporters (GLUTS) in peripheral tissues.

Similarly, Leydig cell hyperplasia is often found in patients with testicular atrophy and androgen insensitivity syndrome[95] and in chronic exposure to toxic chemical agents.[96] Contributory factors in relation to this pathology are reduced testosterone synthesis and impaired regulation of the hypothalamo-gonadal axis with aging (figure 2), decreased sensitivity and numbers of AR, and inhibition of 5α-reductase and aromatase activity.

Such Leydig cell micronodules have been associated with significantly increased total Leydig cell volume and show evidence of functional Leydig cell failure, shown by vacuolization and a decreased T–Leydig cell volume ratio. The T–LH and T–FSH ratios are also significantly decreased, indicating an impaired testicular function at the endocrine as well as the spermatogenic level.[97]

Lifestyle factors in metabolic syndrome and alcoholism cause fibrosis and damage to both pancreatic islets and Leydig cells and can be modified with benefit to both conditions.[98]

New Definition of Androgen Deficiency

This hypothesis leads to a new definition of androgen deficiency in the adult male in accordance with that of diabetes mellitus:

> An absolute or relative deficiency of testosterone or its metabolites according to the needs of that individual at that time in his life.[99]

Terminology

In light of this information, terms like *idiopathic hypergonadotropic hypogonadism* cease to convey meaningful information. Late-onset hypogonadism seems similarly inappropriate because although its symptoms most commonly appear around the age of fifty, it can occur in men in their twenties and thirties, and the gonads may be functioning normally but working against high levels of androgen resistance.

It is suggested that as with diabetes mellitus, the terms *juvenile testosterone deficiency* and *maturity-onset testosterone deficiency* will be more appropriate, as well as using the term *testosterone deficiency syndrome* for the characteristic symptom pattern of androgen deficiency appearing in adult life.

Diagnosis

Like many consensus statements on androgen treatment, the recent Endocrine Society guidelines[100] recommend 'making a diagnosis of androgen deficiency only in men with consistent symptoms and signs and unequivocally low serum testosterone levels' and suggest 'the measurement of morning total testosterone level by a reliable assay as the initial diagnostic test'. However, lower limits of the reference ranges quoted by laboratories in the Eastern United States vary by 350 percent from 4.5 to 15.6 nmol/L (130–450 ng/dL),[101] which is likely to cause confusion in the minds of clinicians trying to establish a definite diagnosis of androgen deficiency.

Because of the high sensitivity but low specificity of questionnaires to detect TDS, the complexity of factors involved in androgen resistance, and the invalidity of androgen assays,[102] it seems logical to adopt the suggestion endorsed by Black et al.,[103] which is that, where typical symptoms or conditions known to be related to androgen deficiency occur, a three-month therapeutic trial of testosterone treatment should be given.

This coincides with the emerging view that 'an emphasis and reliance on serum T alone hinders the clinician's ability to manage testosterone deficiency syndromes (TDS)'.[104] Low total testosterone is just the tip of the iceberg of androgen deficiency.

Treatment

Lacking the equivalent of blood glucose in diabetes to regulate treatment, it is proposed that the sustained remission of symptoms be the guiding factor in regulating treatment, with three to six monthly androgen assays to ensure that physiological levels are maintained, along with safety measurements of PSA and hemoglobin.

Tackling Testosterone Resistance

Since many of the factors causing testosterone resistance are similar to those causing insulin resistance, a similar approach can be used to treating the two conditions either singly or together.

Age and heredity obviously cannot be treated but can help early diagnosis and intervention.

Lifestyle factors such as obesity and, often, associated excess alcohol intake should be intensively treated as the life-threatening factors they are. A diary of food and alcohol intake should be started, and a diet such as the high-protein, low-carbohydrate Atkins diet tried. Exercise should be vigorous but not violent and dynamic, not static. Over the age of fifty, jogging, unless a habit for a number of years, is not recommended. Remember, the grim reaper also wears a tracksuit. If you are severely overweight, swimming is a good form of exercise, and you get double benefit not only from the whole-body exercise but also from losing calories even in comfortably warm water.

Stress can also produce testosterone resistance by causing the release of cortisol, adrenaline, and noradrenaline (epinephrine), which all antagonize testosterone release and action. Easing the load of your life and learning a meditation technique such as mindful meditation can also help greatly.

In conclusion, this evidence-based review of the cellular and molecular mechanisms involved suggests that if a choice has to be made between symptomatology as a whole-body bioassay and standard endocrine measurements in the diagnosis and treatment of androgen deficiency, the seemingly infinite complexities of the actions of these hormones will seem to indicate that the former should take precedence for practical clinical purposes.

Reference for Chapter 3

[1.] H. P. Himsworth, 'Mechanism of Diabetes Mellitus', *The Lancet*, 65 (1939), 118–71.

[2.] A. A. Werner, 'The Male Climacteric: Report of Two Hundred and Seventy-Three Cases', *Journal of the American Medical Association*, 132 (1946), 188–94.

[3.] C. G. Heller and G. B. Myers, 'The Male Climacteric: Its Symptomatology, Diagnosis and Treatment', *Journal of the American Medical Association*, 126 (1944), 472–7.

[4.] T. Reiter, 'Testosterone Implantation: A Clinical Study of 240 Implantations in Ageing Males', *Journal of the American Geriatrics Society*, 11 (1963), 540–50.

[5.] M. Carruthers, *ADAM: Androgen Deficiency in the Adult Male—Causes, Diagnosis and Treatment* (London and New York: Taylor & Francis, 2004).

[6.] R. R. Tremblay and A. J. Morales, 'Canadian Practice Recommendations for Screening, Monitoring and Treating Men Affected by Andropause or Partial Androgen Deficiency', *The Aging Male*, 1 (1998), 213–8.

[7.] L. A. J. Heinemann, T. Zimmermann, A. Vermeulen, C. Thiel, and W. Hummel, 'A New "Aging Males" Symptoms (AMS) Rating Scale', *The Aging Male*, 2 (1999), 105–14.

[8.] C. Kratzik, L. A. Heinemann, F. Saad, D. M. Thai, and E. Rucklinger, 'Composite Screener for Androgen Deficiency Related to the Aging Males' Symptoms Scale', *The Aging Male*, 8 (2005), 157–61.

9. A. Morales, M. Spevack, L. Emerson, I. Kuzmarov, R. Casey, A. Black, and R. Tremblay, 'Adding to the Controversy: Pitfalls in the Diagnosis of Testosterone Deficiency Syndromes with Questionnaires and Biochemistry', *The Aging Male*, 10 (2007), 57–65.

10. G. T'Sjoen, E. Feyen, P. De Kuyper, F. Comhaire, and J. M. Kaufman, 'Self-Referred Patients in an Aging Male Clinic: Much More Than Androgen Deficiency Alone', *The Aging Male*, 6 (2003), 157–65.

11. G. T'Sjoen, S. Goemaere, M. De Meyere, and J. M. Kaufman, 'Perception of Males' Aging Symptoms, Health and Well-Being in Elderly Community-Dwelling Men Is Not Related to Circulating Androgen Levels', *Psychoneuroendocrinology*, 29 (2004), 201–14.

12. J. E. Morley, H. M. Perry III, R. T. Kevorkian, and P. Patrick, 'Comparison of Screening Questionnaires for the Diagnosis of Hypogonadism', *Maturitas*, 53 (2006), 424–9.

13. J. E. Morley, P. Patrick, and H. M. Perry III, 'Evaluation of Assays Available to Measure Free Testosterone', *Metabolism*, 51 (2002), 554–9.

14. Y. Miwa, T. Kaneda, and O. Yokoyama, 'Correlation between the Aging Males' Symptoms Scale and Sex Steroids, Gonadotropins, Dehydroepiandrosterone Sulfate, and Growth Hormone Levels in Ambulatory Men', *The Journal of Sexual Medicine*, 3 (2006), 723–6.

15. T. G. Travison, J. E. Morley, A. B. Araujo, A. B O'Donnel, and J. B. McKinlay, 'The Relationship between Libido and Testosterone Levels in Aging Men', *The Journal of Clinical Endocrinology and Metabolism*, 91 (2006), 2,509–13.

[16.] V. Kupelian, R. Shabsigh, T. G. Travison, S. T. Page, A. B. Araujo, and J. B. McKinlay, 'Is There a Relationship between Sex Hormones and Erectile Dysfunction? Results from the Massachusetts Male Aging Study', *The Journal of Urology*, 176 (2006), 2,584–8.

[17.] A. B. Araujo, G. R. Esche, V. Kupelian, A. B. O'donnell, T. G. Travison, R. E. Williams, R. V. Clark, and J. B. McKinlay, 'Prevalence of Symptomatic Androgen Deficiency in Men', *The Journal of Clinical Endocrinology and Metabolism*, 92 (2007), 4,241–7.

[18.] M. Zitzmann, S. Faber, and E. Nieschlag, 'Association of Specific Symptoms and Metabolic Risks with Serum Testosterone in Older Men', *The Journal of Clinical Endocrinology and Metabolism*, 91 (2006), 4,335–43.

[19.] L. Reyes-Vallejo, S. Lazarou, and A. Morgentaler, 'Subjective Sexual Response to Testosterone Replacement Therapy Based on Initial Serum Levels of Total Testosterone', *The Journal of Sexual Medicine*, 4/1 (2007), 757–62.

[20.] S. Kelleher, A. J. Conway, and D. J. Handelsman, 'Blood Testosterone Threshold for Androgen Deficiency Symptoms', *The Journal of Clinical Endocrinology and Metabolism*, 89/3 (2004), 813–7.

[21.] A. J. Conway, D. J. Handelsman, D. W. Lording, B. Stuckey, and J. D. Zajac, 'Use, Misuse and Abuse of Androgens: The Endocrine Society of Australia Consensus Guidelines for Androgen Prescribing', *Medical Journal of Australia*, 172 (2000), 220–4.

[22.] E. Nieschlag, R. Swerdloff, H. M. Behre, L. J. Gooren, J. M. Kaufman, J. J. Legros, B. Lunenfeld, J. E. Morley, C. Schulman, C. Wang, W. Weidner, and F. C. Wu, 'Investigation, Treatment and

Monitoring of Late-Onset Hypogonadism in Males: ISA, ISSAM, and EAU Recommendations', *The Aging Male*, 8 (2005), 56–8.

23. S. Bhasin, G. R. Cunningham, F. J. Hayes, A. M. Matsumoto, P. J. Snyder, R. S. Swerdloff, et al., 'Testosterone Therapy in Adult Men with Androgen Deficiency Syndromes: An Endocrine Society Clinical Practice Guideline', *The Journal of Clinical Endocrinology and Metabolism*, 9/1 (2006), 995–2,010.

24. M. Carruthers, T. R. Trinick, and M. J. Wheeler, 'The Validity of Androgen Assays', *The Aging Male*, 10 (2007), 165–72.

25. S. Nussey and S. A. Whitehead, *Endocrinology: An Integrated Approach* (Oxford: BIOS Scientific Publishers Ltd, 2001).

26. J. M. Kaufman and A. Vermeulen, 'Androgens in Male Senescence', In E. Nieschlag and H. M. Behre, eds., *Testosterone: Action, Deficiency, Substitution* (Berlin: Springer Verlag, 1998), 437–71.

27. A. Vermeulen, 'Declining Androgens with Age: An Overview', In B. Oddens and A. Vermeulen, eds., *Androgens and the Aging Male* (New York, NY: The Parthenon Publishing Group, 1996), 3–14.

28. H. A. Feldman, C. Longcope, C. A. Derby, C. B. Johannes, A. B. Araujo, A. D. Coviello, W. J. Bremner, and J. B. McKinlay, 'Age Trends in the Level of Serum Testosterone and Other Hormones in Middle-Aged Men: Longitudinal Results from the Massachusetts Male Aging Study', *The Journal of Clinical Endocrinology and Metabolism*, 87 (2002), 589–98.

29. B. A. Mohr, A. T. Guay, A. B. O'Donnell, and J. B. McKinlay, 'Normal, Bound and Nonbound Testosterone Levels in Normally Ageing Men: Results from the Massachusetts Male Aging Study', *Clinical Endocrinology* (Oxford), 62 (2005), 64–73.

30. T. G. Travison, A. B. Araujo, A. B. O'Donnell, V. Kupelian, and J. B. McKinlay. 'A Population-Level Decline in Serum Testosterone Levels in American Men', *The Journal of Clinical Endocrinology and Metabolism*, 92 (2007), 196–202.

31. S. R. Plymate, J. S. Tenover, and W. J. Bremner, 'Circadian Variation in Testosterone, Sex Hormone-Binding Globulin, and Calculated Non-Sex Hormone-Binding Globulin Bound Testosterone in Healthy Young and Elderly Men', *Journal of Andrology*, 10 (1989), 366–71.

32. M. J. Diver, K. E. Imtiaz, A. M. Ahmad, J. P. Vora, and W. D. Fraser, 'Diurnal Rhythms of Serum Total, Free and Bioavailable Testosterone and of SHBG in Middle-Aged Men Compared with Those in Young Men', *Clinical Endocrinology* (Oxford), 58 (2003), 710–7.

33. P. Y. Takahashi, P. Votruba, M. Abu-Rub, K. Mielke, and J. D. Veldhuis, 'Age Attenuates Testosterone Secretion Driven by Amplitude-Varying Pulses of Recombinant Human Luteinizing Hormone during Acute Gonadotrope Inhibition in Healthy Men', *The Journal of Clinical Endocrinology and Metabolism*, 92 (2007), 3,626–32.

34. W. B. Neaves, L. Johnson, J. C. Porter, C. R. Parker Jr, and C. S. Petty, 'Leydig Cell Numbers, Daily Sperm Production, and Serum Gonadotropin Levels in Aging Men', *The Journal of Clinical Endocrinology and Metabolism*, 59 (1984), 756–63.

35. L. Gnessi, A. Fabbri, and G. Spera, 'Gonadal Peptides as Mediators of Development and Functional Control of the Testis: An Integrated System with Hormones and Local Environment', *Endocrine Reviews*, 18 (1997), 541–609.

[36.] G. F. Weinbauer, J. Gromoll, M. Simoni, and E. Nieschlag, 'Physiology of Testicular Function', in E. Nieschlag and H. Behre, eds., *Andrology: Male Reproductive Health and Dysfunction* (Berlin: Springer, 1997), 25–57.

[37.] V. P. Shanbhag and R. Sodergard, 'The Temperature Dependence of the Binding of 5-Alpha Dihydrotestosterone, Testosterone and Estradiol to the Sex Hormone Globulin (SHBG) of Human Plasma', *Journal of Steroid Biochemistry*, 24 (1986), 549–55.

[38.] L. Bujan, M. Daudin, J. P. Charlet, P. Thonneau, and R. Mieusset, 'Increase in Scrotal Temperature in Car Drivers', *Human Reproduction*, 15 (2000), 1,355–7.

[39.] M. Carruthers, *ADAM: Androgen Deficiency in the Adult Male—Causes, Diagnosis and Treatment* (London and New York: Taylor & Francis, 2004).

[40.] L. Gandini, P. Sgro, F. Lombardo, D. Paoli, F. Culasso, T. Toselli, P. Tsamatropoulos, and A. Lenzi, 'Effect of Chemo or Radiotherapy on Sperm Parameters of Testicular Cancer Patients', *Human Reproduction*, 21 (2006), 2,882–9.

[41.] A. W. Meikle, D. T. Bishop, J. D. Stringham, and D. W. West, 'Quantitating Genetic and Non-Genetic Gactors to Determine Plasma Sex Steroid Variation in Normal Male Twins', *Metabolism*, 35 (1987), 1,090–5.

[42.] J. M. Kaufman and A. Vermeulen, 'Androgens in Male Senescence', in E. Nieschlag and H. M. Behre, eds., *Testosterone: Action, Deficiency, Substitution* (Berlin: Springer Verlag, 1998), 437–71.

[43.] E. Hogervorst, J. Williams, M. Budge, L. Barnetson, M. Combrinck, and A. D. Smith, 'Serum Total Testosterone Is Lower in Men with Alzheimer's Disease', *Neuroendocrinology Letters*, 22 (2001), 163–8.

[44.] O. Elwan, M. Abdallah, I. Issa, Y. Taher, and M. Tamawy, 'Hormonal Changes in Cerebral Infarction in the Young and Elderly', *Journal of the Neurological Sciences*, 98 (1990), 235–43.

[45.] M. S. Okun, W. M. McDonald, and M. R. DeLong, 'Refractory Nonmotor Symptoms in Male Patients with Parkinson's Disease Due to Testosterone Deficiency: A Common Unrecognized Comorbidity', *Archives of Neurology*, 59 (2002), 807–11.

[46.] K. Christiansen, 'Behavioural Correlates of Testosterone', in E. Nieschlag and H. M. Behre, eds., *Testosterone: Action, Deficiency, Substitution* (Berlin: Springer Verlag, 1998), 107–42.

[47.] P. K. Opstad, 'Androgenic Hormones During Prolonged Physical Stress, Sleep, and Energy Deficiency', *The Journal of Clinical Endocrinology and Metabolism*, 74 (1992), 1,176–83.

[48.] Ibid.

[49.] Q. Dong, F. Hawker, D. McWilliam, M. Bangah, H. Burger, and D. J. Handelsman, 'Circulating Immunoreactive Inhibin and Testosterone Levels in Men with Critical Illness', *Clinical Endocrinology*, 36 (1992), 399–404.

[50.] D. Sparrow, R. Bosse, and J. W. Rowe, 'The Influence of Age, Alcohol Consumption, and Body Build on Gonadal Function in Men', *The Journal of Clinical Endocrinology and Metabolism*, 51 (1980), 508–12.

[51.] F. M. Badr, A. Bartke, S. Dalterio, and W. Bulger, 'Suppression of Testosterone Production by Ethyl Alcohol: Possible Mode of Action', *Steroids*, 30 (1977), 647–55.

[52.] V. Rettori and S. M. McCann, 'Role of Nitric Oxide and Alcohol on Gonadotropin Release in Vitro and in Vivo', *Annals of the New York Academy of Sciences*, 840 (1998), 185–93.

[53.] J. Wright, 'Endocrine Effects of Alcohol', *Journal of Clinical Endocrinology and Metabolism*, 7 (1978), 351–67.

[54.] E. K. Hamalainen, H. Adlercreutz, P. Puska, and P. Pietinen, 'Decrease of Serum Total and Free Testosterone during a Low-Fat High-Fibre Diet', *Journal of Steroid Biochemistry and Molecular Biology*, 18 (1983), 369–70.

[55.] Ibid.

[56.] G. Corona, E. Mannucci, A. D. Fisher, F. Lotti, V. Ricca, G. Balercia, L. Petrone, G. Forti, and M. Maggi, 'Effect of Hyperprolactinemia in Male Patients Consulting for Sexual Dysfunction', *The Journal of Sexual Medicine*, 4 (2007), 1,485–93.

[57.] T. Schurmeyer and E. Nieschlag, 'Effect of Ketoconazole and Other Imidazole Fungicides on Testosterone Biosynthesis', *Acta Endocrinologica* (Copenhagen), 105 (1984), 275– 80.

[58.] E. A. Greco, M. Pili, R. Bruzziches, G. Corona, G. Spera, and A. Aversa, 'Testosterone: Estradiol Ratio Changes Associated with Long-Term Tadalafil Administration: A Pilot Study', *The Journal of Sexual Medicine*, 3 (2006), 716–22.

[59.] T. Misugi, K. Ozaki, K. El Beltagy, O. Tokuyama, K. Honda, and O. Ishiko, 'Insulin-Lowering Agents Inhibit Synthesis of Testosterone in Ovaries of DHEA-Induced PCOS Rats', *Gynecologic and Obstetric Investigation*, 61 (2006), 208–15.

[60.] H. M. Garmes, M. A. Tambascia, and D.E. Zantut-Wittmann, 'Endocrine-Metabolic Effects of the Treatment with Pioglitazone in Obese Patients with Polycystic Ovary Syndrome', *Gynecological Endocrinology*, 21 (2005), 317–23.

61. S. E. Nissen and K. Wolski, 'Effect of Rosiglitazone on the Risk of Myocardial Infarction and Death from Cardiovascular Causes', *New England Journal of Medicine*, 356 (2007), 2,457–71.

62. W. M. Pardridge, 'Transport of Protein-Bound Hormones into Tissues in Vivo', *Endocrine Reviews*, 2 (1981), 103–23.

63. C. Longcope, H. A. Feldman, J. B. McKinlay, and A. B. Araujo, 'Diet and Sex Hormone-Binding Globulin', *The Journal of Clinical Endocrinology and Metabolism*, 85 (2000), 293–6.

64. D. C. Anderson, 'Sex-Hormone-Binding Globulin', *Journal of Clinical Endocrinology and Metabolism*, 3 (1974), 69–96.

65. D. J. Hryb, A. M. Nakhla, S. M. Kahn, J. St George, N. C. Levy, N. A. Romas, and W. Rosner, 'Sex Hormone-Binding Globulin in the Human Prostate Is Locally Synthesized and May Act as an Autocrine/Paracrine Effector', *Journal of Biology Chemistry*, 277 (2002), 26,618–22.

66. W. Rosner, D. J. Hryb, M. S. Khan, A. M. Nakhla, and N. A. Romas, 'Androgen and Estrogen Signaling at the Cell Membrane via G-Proteins and Cyclic Adenosine Monophosphate', *Steroids*, 64 (1999), 100–6.

67. S. M. Kahn, D. J. Hryb, A. M. Nakhla, N. A. Romas, and W. Rosner, 'Sex Hormone-Binding Globulin Is Synthesized in Target Cells', *Journal of Endocrinology*, 175 (2002), 113–20.

68. N. Fortunati, 'Sex Hormone-Binding Globulin: Not Only a Transport Protein. What News Is around the Corner?', *Journal of Endocrinological Investigation*, 22 (1999), 223–34.

69. A. M. Traish and N. Kim, 'Weapons of Penile Smooth Muscle Destruction: Androgen Deficiency Promotes Accumulation of Adipocytes in the Corpus Cavernosum', *The Aging Male*, 8 (2005), 141–6.

70. A. M. Traish and A. T. Guay, 'Are Androgens Critical for Penile Erections in Humans? Examining the Clinical and Preclinical Evidence', *The Journal of Sexual Medicine*, 3 (2006), 382–404.

71. D. Kapoor, E. Goodwin, K. S. Channer, and T. H. Jones, 'Testosterone Replacement Therapy Improves Insulin Resistance, Glycaemic Control, Visceral Adiposity and Hypercholesterolaemia in Hypogonadal Men with Type 2 Diabetes', *European Journal of Endocrinology*, 154 (2006), 899–906.

72. A. A. Yassin, F. Saad, and A Traish, 'Testosterone Undecanoate Restores Erectile Function in a Subset of Patients With Venous Leakage: A Series of Case Reports', *The Journal of Sexual Medicine*, 3 (2006), 727–35.

73. A. A. Yassin and F. Saad, 'Improvement of Sexual Function in Men with Late-Onset Hypogonadism Treated with Testosterone Only', *The Journal of Sexual Medicine*, 4 (2007), 497–501.

74. A. Aversa, A. M. Isidori, M. U. De Martino, M. Caprio, E. Fabbrini, M. Rocchietti-March, G. Frajese, and A. Fabbri, 'Androgens and Penile Erection: Evidence for a Direct Relationship between Free Testosterone and Cavernous Vasodilation in Men with Erectile Dysfunction', *Clinical Endocrinology* (Oxford), 53 (2000), 517–22.

75. A. Aversa, A. M. Isidori, G. Spera, A. Lenzi, and A. Fabbri, 'Androgens Improve Cavernous Vasodilation and Response to Sildenafil in Patients with Erectile Dysfunction', *Clinical Endocrinology* (Oxford), 58 (2003), 632–8.

76. N. Gonzalez-Cadavid, D. Vernet, A. Fuentes Navarro, J. A. Rodriguez, R. S. Swerdloff, and J. Rajfer, 'Up-Regulation of the Levels of Androgen Receptor and Its mRNA by Androgens in Smooth-Muscle Cells from Rat Penis', *Molecular and Cellular Endocrinology*, 90 (1993), 219–29.

77. R. W. Lewis and T. M. Mills, 'Effect of Androgens on Penile Tissue', *Endocrine*, 23 (2004), 101–5.

78. A. A. Yassin and F. Saad, 'Improvement of Sexual Function in Men with Late-Onset Hypogonadism Treated with Testosterone Only', *The Journal of Sexual Medicine*, 4 (2007), 497–501.

79. E. A. Greco, G. Spera, and A. Aversa, 'Combining Testosterone and PDE5 Inhibitors in Erectile Dysfunction: Basic Rationale and Clinical Evidences', *European Urology*, 50 (2006), 940–7.

80. A. M. Traish, I. Goldstein, and N. N. Kim, 'Testosterone and Erectile Function: From Basic Research to a New Clinical Paradigm for Managing Men with Androgen Insufficiency and Erectile Dysfunction', *European Urology*, 52 (2007), 54–70.

81. L. Vignozzi, A. Morelli, S. Filippi, S. Ambrosini, R. Mancina, M. Luconi, S. Mungai, G. B. Vannelli, X. H. Zhang, G. Forti, and M. Maggi, 'Testosterone Regulates RhoA/Rho-Kinase Signaling in Two Distinct Animal Models of Chemical Diabetes', *The Journal of Sexual Medicine*, 4 (2007), 620–30.

82. N. Pitteloud, V. K. Mootha, A. A. Dwyer, M. Hardin, H. Lee, K. F. Eriksson, D. Tripathy, M. Yialamas, L. Groop, D. Elahi, and F. J. Hayes, 'Relationship between Testosterone Levels, Insulin Sensitivity, and Mitochondrial Function in Men', *Diabetes Care*, 28 (2005), 1,636–42.

83. J. B. Kostis, G. Jackson, R. Rosen, E. Barrett-Connor, K. Billups, A. L. Burnett, C. Carson III, M. Cheitlin, R. DeBusk, V. Fonseca, P. Ganz, I. Goldstein, A. Guay, D. Hatzichristou, J. E. Hollander, A. Hutter, S. Katz, R. A. Kloner, M. Mittleman, F. Montorsi, P. Montorsi, A. Nehra, R. Sadovsky, and R. Shabsigh, 'Sexual Dysfunction and Cardiac Risk (The Second Princeton Consensus Conference)', *American Journal of Cardiology*, 96 (2005), 313–21.

84. G. M. Rosano, I. Sheiban, R. Massaro, P. Pagnotta, G. Marazzi, C. Vitale, G. Mercuro, M. Volterrani, A. Aversa, and M. Fini, 'Low Testosterone Levels Are Associated with Coronary Artery Disease in Male Patients with Angina', *International Journal of Impotence Research*, 19 (2007), 176–82.

85. D. O. Hardy, H. I. Scher, T. Bogenreider, P. Sabbatini, Z. F. Zhang, D. M. Nanus, and J. F. Catterall, 'Androgen Receptor CAG Repeat Lengths in Prostate Cancer: Correlation with Age of Onset', *The Journal of Clinical Endocrinology and Metabolism*, 81 (1996), 4,400–5.

86. P. Crabbe, V. Bogaert, D. De Bacquer, S. Goemaere, H. Zmierczak, and J. M. Kaufman, 'Part of the Interindividual Variation in Serum Testosterone Levels in Healthy Men Reflects Differences in Androgen Sensitivity and Feedback Setpoint: Contribution of the Androgen Receptor Polyglutamine Tract Polymorphism', *The Journal of Clinical Endocrinology and Metabolism*, 92 (2007), 3,604–10.

87. Y. Ruhayel, K. Lundin, Y. Giwercman, C. Hallden, M. Willen, and A. Giwercman, 'Androgen Receptor Gene GGN and CAG Polymorphisms among Severely Oligozoospermic and Azoospermic Swedish Men', *Human Reproduction*, 19 (2004), 2,076–83.

88. E. L. Aschim, A. Nordenskjold, A. Giwercman, K. B. Lundin, Y. Ruhayel, T. B. Haugen, T. Grotmol, and Y. L. Giwercman, 'Linkage between Cryptorchidism, Hypospadias, and GGN Repeat Length in the Androgen Receptor Gene', *The Journal of Clinical Endocrinology and Metabolism*, 89 (2004), 5,105–9.

89. K. B. Lundin, A. Giwercman, N. Dizeyi, and Y. L. Giwercman, 'Functional in Vitro Characterisation of the Androgen Receptor GGN Polymorphism', Molecular and Cellular Endocrinology, 264 (2007), 184–7.

90. M. Zitzmann and E. Nieschlag, 'The CAG Repeat Polymorphism within the Androgen Receptor Gene and Maleness', International Journal of Andrology, 26 (2003), 76–83.

91. A. S. Om and K. W. Chung, 'Dietary Zinc Deficiency Alters 5 Alpha-Reduction and Aromatization of Testosterone and Androgen and Estrogen Receptors in Rat Liver', *Journal of Nutrition*, 126 (1996), 842–8.

92. C. P. Cardozo, C. Michaud, M. C. Ost, A. E. Fliss, E. Yang, C. Patterson, S. J. Hall, and A. J. Caplan, 'C-Terminal Hsp-Interacting Protein Slows Androgen Receptor Synthesis and Reduces Its Rate of Degradation', Archives of Biochemistry and Biophysics, 410 (2003), 134–40.

93. S. McDonald, L. Brive, D. B. Agus, H. I. Scher, and K. R. Ely, 'Ligand Responsiveness in Human Prostate Cancer: Structural Analysis of Mutant Androgen Receptors from LNCaP and CWR22 Tumors', *Cancer Research*, 60 (2000), 2,317–22.

94. M. Fu, M. Rao, C. Wang, T. Sakamaki, J. Wang, D. Di Vizio, X. Zhang, C. Albanese, S. Balk, C. Chang, S. Fan, E. Rosen, J. J. Palvimo, O. A. Janne, S. Muratoglu, M. L. Avantaggiati, and R. G.

Pestell, 'Acetylation of Androgen Receptor Enhances Coactivator Binding and Promotes Prostate Cancer Cell Growth', Molecular and Cellular Biology, 23 (2003), 8,563–75.

95. M. Holm, E. Rajpert-De Meyts, A. M. Andersson, and N. E. Skakkebaek, 'Leydig Cell Micronodules Are a Common Finding in Testicular Biopsies from Men with Impaired Spermatogenesis and Are Associated with Decreased Testosterone/LH Ratio', The Journal of Pathology, 199 (2003), 378–86.

96. E. D. Clegg, J. C. Cook, R. E. Chapin, P. M. Foster, and G. P. Daston, 'Leydig Cell Hyperplasia and Adenoma Formation: Mechanisms and Relevance to Humans', Reproductive Toxicology, 11 (1997), 107–21.

97. M. Holm, E. Rajpert-De Meyts, A. M. Andersson, and N. E. Skakkebaek, 'Leydig Cell Micronodules Are a Common Finding in Testicular Biopsies from Men with Impaired Spermatogenesis and Are Associated with Decreased Testosterone/LH Ratio', The Journal of Pathology, 199 (2003), 378–86.

98. A. B. Araujo, G. R. Esche, V. Kupelian, A. B. O'donnell, T. G. Travison, R. E. Williams, R. V. Clark, and J. B. McKinlay, 'Prevalence of Symptomatic Androgen Deficiency in Men', The Journal of Clinical Endocrinology and Metabolism, 92 (2007), 4,241–7.

99. M. Carruthers, ADAM: Androgen deficiency in the Adult Male— Causes, Diagnosis and Treatment (London and New York: Taylor & Francis, 2004).

100. S. Bhasin, G. R. Cunningham, F. J. Hayes, A. M. Matsumoto, P. J. Snyder, R. S. Swerdloff, et al., 'Testosterone Therapy in Adult Men with Androgen Deficiency Syndromes: An Endocrine Society

Clinical Practice Guideline', *The Journal of Clinical Endocrinology and Metabolism*, 91 (2006), 1,995–2,010.

[101.] S. Lazarou, L. Reyes-Vallejo, and A. Morgentaler, 'Wide Variability in Laboratory Reference Values for Serum Testosterone', *The Journal of Sexual Medicine*, 3 (2006), 1,085–9.

[102.] M. Carruthers, T. R. Trinick, and M. J. Wheeler, 'The Validity of Androgen Assays', *The Aging Male*, 10 (2007), 165–72.

[103.] A. M. Black, A. G. Day, and A. Morales, 'The Reliability of Clinical and Biochemical Assessment in Symptomatic Late-Onset Hypogonadism: Can a Case Be Made for a 3-Month Therapeutic Trial?', *BJU International*, 94 (2004), 1,066–70.

[104.] A. Morales, M. Spevack, L. Emerson, I. Kuzmarov, R. Casey, A. Black, and R. Tremblay, 'Adding to the Controversy: Pitfalls in the Diagnosis of Testosterone Deficiency Syndromes with Questionnaires and Biochemistry', *The Aging Male*, 10 (2007), 57–65.

Chapter 4
Sources of External Resistance

The greater the ignorance the greater the dogmatism

Osler

Medical Orthodoxy

With the motto 'Firstly, do no harm' and a five- or six-year training program before they are let loose to the public, as well as another five- or six-year postgraduate program before they are expected to practice as independent specialists, it is unsurprising that doctors seldom think for themselves. Instead, their thought and deeds tend to be prescribed for them by their peers and seniors, often in the form of consensus and guidelines. These are sent down as from oracular beings usually in the form of peer-reviewed article in leading journals.

You can tell it is a leading journal by its impact factor, which ranges from the top, holy writ of the *New England Journal of Medicine* at 50 in general medicine to the other American heavyweight *Journal of the American Medical Journal*, at 30, with most specialist journals weighing in at a puny 3-4. In the UK, as in America, there are two big ones, *The Lancet* at 39, and the *British Medical Journal* at only 16.

Also, these journals like to blow their own trumpets and make headlines in the newspapers and media by having well-oiled publicity machines to announce their latest papers to both doctors and the general public. These pronouncements are amplified by the relevant pharmaceutical companies if they are favorable and are played down by hired guns of experts with opposing views if they are unfavorable. This can and does lead to a bias toward eminence-based medicine rather than evidenced-based medicine.

As for the young researcher, it is a question of publish or perish, and your next research grant may depend on singing a popular song, while thinking outside the box is not encouraged. This can endanger your career, your job prospects, and your research grants and even get you struck off the medical register and stopped from practicing if your ideas are sufficiently unorthodox and heretical. This is the equivalent of being excommunicated from the church if you are judged a radical priest. It forms a strong tide of medical opinion if you choose to swim against it. To give you some idea of how strong, I have done an analysis of articles appearing in both the leading medical journals in the USA and UK.

Another impediment to a balanced evaluation of the literature is that these leading journals usually don't provide abstracts on any of the search databases so that the pronouncements only come down from the Olympic heights of academia translated by medical journalists or press releases to newspapers. This results in extensive filtering of messages and considerable difficulty and expense if you wish to analyze the original paper.

To get a general impression where peer pressure is firmly pointing the general physician, let's take a look at references to testosterone in the leading journals in general medicine in the USA and UK during the last fifteen years.

New England Journal of Medicine (Impact Factor: 54)

Remarkably, only three references have been found to testosterone treatment and except for the third carried a generally negative message.

Articles

1. Basaria, S.; Coviello, A.d., Travison, T.g. et al (27 authors)'Adverse Events Associated with Testosterone Administration'363(2010)1-14.

2. Swerloff, R. Anawalth, b.d., 'Testosterone replacement therapy' New Engl.J.Med 371/21(2014) 2032-2034. (Poll coming out against but complaints of jury rigging by opponents of TRT)

3. 3. Snyder PJ, Bhasin S, Cunningham GR, Matsumoto AM, Stephens-Shields AJ, Cauley JA et al. (33Authors) 'Effects of Testosterone Treatment in Older Men.'374/7 (2016);):611-624.(First 3 of 7 NIH funded studies)

Letters: 0

Journal of the American Medical Association (Impact Factor: 30)
Articles and Editorials

1. Basaria, S., 'Testosterone Levels for Evaluation of Androgen Deficiency', *JAMA*, 313/17 (2015), 1,749–1,750. (Attempting the impossible).

2. Garnick, M. B., 'Testosterone Replacement Therapy Faces FDA Scrutiny', *JAMA, 313/6* (2015), 563–564. (Generally negative.)

3. Morgentaler, A., Traish, A., and Kacker, R., 'Deaths and Cardiovascular Events)) in Men *Rece*iving Testosterone', *JAMA*, 311/9 (2014), 961–962. (A powerful and positive voice but only in a letter.)

4. Vigen, R., O'Donnell, C. I., Baron, A. E., Grunwald, G. K., Maddox, T. M., Bradley, S. M., et al., 'Association of Testosterone Therapy with Mortality, Myocardial

Infarction, and Stroke in Men with Low Testosterone Levels', *JAMA*, 310/17 (2013), 1,829–1,836. (A large negative article which had twisted statistics and should have been withdrawn.)

5. Bhasin, S., Travison, T. G., Storer, T. W., Lakshman, K., Kaushik, M., Mazer, N. A., et al., 'Effect of Testosterone Supplementation with and without a Dual 5-Alpha-Reductase Inhibitor on Fat-Free Mass in Men with Suppressed Testosterone Production: A Randomized Controlled Trial', *JAMA*, 307/9 (2012), 931–939. (Generally negative article.)

6. Emmelot-Vonk, M. H., Verhaar, H. J., Nakhai Pour, H. R., Aleman, A., Lock, T. M., Bosch, J. L., et al., 'Effect of Testosterone Supplementation on Functional Mobility, Cognition, and Other Parameters in Older Men: A Randomized Controlled Trial', *JAMA*, 299/1 (2008), 39–52. (Generally negative article focusing on a few effects.)

7. Marks, L. S., Mazer, N. A., Mostaghel, E., Hess, D. L., Dorey, F. J., Epstein, J. I., et al., 'Effect of Testosterone Replacement Therapy on Prostate Tissue in Men with Late-Onset Hypogonadism: A Randomized Controlled Trial', *JAMA*, 296/19 (2006), 2,351–2,361. (More-balanced article.)

8. Ding, E. L., Song, Y., Malik, V. S., and Liu, S., 'Sex Differences of Endogenous Sex Hormones and Risk of Type 2 Diabetes: A Systematic Review and Meta-Analysis', *JAMA*, 295/11 (2006), 1,288–1,299.

9. Bhasin, S., Storer, T. W., Javanbakht, M., Berman, N., Yarasheski, K. E., Phillips, J., et al., 'Testosterone Replacement and Resistance Exercise in HIV-Infected Men with Weight Loss and Low Testosterone Levels', *JAMA*, 283/6 (2000), 763–770.

Letters

1. Morgentaler, A., Traish, A., and Kacker, R., 'Deaths and Cardiovascular Events in Men Receiving Testosterone', *JAMA*, 311/9 (2014), 961–962. (A powerful and positive voice but only in a letter.)

Britsh Journals

Lancet

Articles

1. Basaria, S., 'Male Hypogonadism', *Lancet*, 383/9,924 (2014), 1,250–1,263.

2. Page, S. T., 'Testosterone, Cardiovascular Disease, and Mortality in Men: Living in the Dark', *Lancet Diabetes and Endocrinology*, 2/8 (2014) 609–611.

3. Harris, O. L., 'FDA Declines Approval of Testosterone Drug for Third Time', *Lancet Diabetes and Endocrinology*, 1/1 (2013), 14.

4. Vigano, A., Piccioni, M., Trutschnigg, B., Hornby, L., Chaudhury, P., and Kilgour, R., 'Male Hypogonadism Associated with Advanced Cancer: A Systematic Review', *Lancet Oncology*, 11/7 (2010), 679–684.

5. Sjoqvist, F., Garle, M., and Rane, A., 'Use of Doping Agents, Particularly Anabolic Steroids, in Sports and Society', *Lancet*, 371/9,627 (2008), 1,872–1,882.

6. Lawrence, D., 'US Panel Urges Caution on Testosterone Therapy: Large-Scale Trials of Efficacy and Safety Are Needed before Widespread Use Can Be Recommended', *Lancet*, 362/9,397 (2003), 1,725.

The BMJ

Articles

1. Wolfe, S. M., 'Increased Heart Attacks in Men Using Testosterone: The UK Importantly Lags Far Behind the US in Prescribing Testosterone, *The BMJ*, 348 (2014), 1,789. (Commissioned article—very negative.)

Letters

1. Gorricho, J., Gavilan, E., and Gervas, J., 'Marketing, Not Evidence Based Arguments, Has Probably Increased Testosterone Prescribing', *The BMJ*, 345 (2012), e6905.

2. Hackett, G., Kirby, M., Jackson, G., and Wylie, K., 'Evidenced Medicine Inevitably Increases Testosterone Prescribing', *The BMJ*, 345 (2012), e6167.

3. Gan, E. H., Pattman, S., Pearce, S., and Quinton, R., 'Many Men Are Receiving Unnecessary Testosterone Prescriptions', *The BMJ*, 345 (2012), e5469.

4. Delamothe, T., 'Monkey Business: Reflections on Testosterone', *The BMJ*, 345 (2012) e4967.

5. Kermode-Scott, B., 'Canadian Regulators Dismiss Complaint about Campaign Publicizing Low Testosterone', *The BMJ*, 343 (2011), d5501.

6. Kmietowicz, Z., 'New UK Guidelines Highlight Role of Testosterone in Sexual Disorders', *The BMJ*, 341 (2010), c5305.

7. Spence, D., 'Men Behaving Madly: Testosterone Replacement Therapy', *The BMJ*, 340 (2010), c1493.

8. Stone, J. A., 'Testosterone Supplementation: An Unfortunate Juxtaposition', *The BMJ*, 336/7,638 (2008), 234.

What can we conclude from this brief survey of the literature? What is the general physician treating middle-aged men that is reading one or more of these journals supposed to learn from them about the importance or safety of testosterone treatment?

Most of them will be looking at the infrequency of articles on the subject and concluding that testosterone deficiency is an uncommon condition, difficult to establish, highly controversial, and probably dangerous to treat. They will probably think it may be best left to endocrinologists, who are supposed to be the experts in such things.

While up to 10 percent of men with symptoms of testosterone deficiency in the USA get treated, in the UK, sales of testosterone have been flat-lining over the last ten years, and less than 2 percent of the 20 percent of men over the age of fifty with the highly characteristic symptoms are being treated. Because of the difficulty in getting testosterone treatment from a general practitioner in the UK particularly, a high proportion of cases with symptoms and related conditions such as diabetes go untreated or is forced to go privately or enter 'the loop'.

This is where the patient feels that, with the onset of the typical symptoms confirmed by a questionnaire such as the aging male symptom scale on the website of a private clinic specializing in testosterone treatment, he must insist on having the testosterone level in his blood measured. It is usually reported erroneously as being within the normal range. If the patient persists, he is referred, usually after a waiting period of two to three months or longer, to an endocrinologist, who is equally likely to miss the diagnosis and refuse a therapeutic trial of treatment, referring him back round the loop to his general practitioner, who is not allowed to prescribe testosterone without the specialist's say-so even if he believes it may help. In what other field of medicine is such a sorry state of affairs allowed to continue even with the apparent backing of orthodox medical opinion as reflected in the journals?

How can we overcome the problems of orthodoxy in the medical profession? This is the central problem that I and my friends and colleagues in organizations such as the Society for the Study of Testosterone Deficiency have been tackling by getting articles published over the past fifteen years and holding international conferences with speakers from all over the world describing the effectiveness and safety of testosterone treatment. These conferences have been reported, and the last one has been made available as a webcast on our website, www. testosteronedeficiency.org. There, free of charge, anyone can see the leading international speakers from the UK, USA, Australia, Russia, and Scandinavia talking about the latest advances in testosterone treatment and discussing the key papers in the field (www.andropause.org.uk).

Hyper-regulation

Both in the USA and now the UK, medico-legal concerns are playing a larger part in day-to-day medical practice. Not for nothing has there appeared in the USA bumper stickers saying 'Become a doctor and support two lawyers'.

People seem to think that you can legislate for a cure. You have a right to the best treatment that your doctor knows how to provide, but there are risks to all treatments, even aspirin, which can make you bleed to death. Risk assessment is a difficult pastime, and while side effects can be classified as common, less common, and rare, the individuals who get them increasingly often feel aggrieved and look around for someone to sue. Unfortunately, while you can expect the pharmaceutical companies to do all reasonable tests on animals and humans and that medicines will be prescribed appropriately and expertly, nothing is absolutely safe in medicine.

We are therefore breeding a generation of doctors who are willing to do less and less for fear of being sued—what I call the do-little doctors. Rather than adopt the motto 'Firstly, do no harm', their motto is 'Firstly, take no chances'. Bold is bad! Like surgeons, there are a few old doctors, a few bold doctors, but very few old-bold doctors.

Carried to extremes, this can severely limit the range of treatments they are willing to prescribe, especially when it comes to the limits of orthodox medicine and preventive medicine they are willing to undertake. Don't stick your neck out, or your head may be chopped off by the insurers or one of the regulatory bodies. The dead hand of regulatory medicine is tightening its grip on the steering wheel of medical practice all the time.

This is an offshoot of orthodoxy and is one of the suckers strangling the tree of medical knowledge. It is used for two main purposes, firstly, by self-styled experts to maintain their status by dictating how other doctors should practice and, secondly, in a futile attempt to gain control of the spiraling costs of medicine. This is a false economy in the case of artificially limiting testosterone use, leaving symptomatic men untreated, and the severe conditions in which testosterone deficiency plays a major role, such as diabetes, go unchecked.

While some guidelines are essential in many fields of medicine, when they become inflexible rules which allow for no individual variation in clinical practice according to experience, they become a hindrance and limitation on a doctor's ability to provide the best medicine according to his or her experience. An extreme example of this is the Australian situation of laying down a threshold of 6 nmol/L (176 ng/dL) total testosterone above which no man is supposed to receive TRT under the state benefits system.

This is not science; it is nonsense. Labs differ, methods differ, and interpretation of so-called normal ranges differ.[1] Sampling conditions differ, levels of testosterone in nonfasting samples being up to 30 percent lower than fasting. According to his testosterone receptors, every man has his own optimal range for according to his age, level of activity, and performance together with the sensitivity or resistance of his androgen receptors. Finally, there is the killer point that there is no relationship between the testosterone level in the blood and the symptoms of testosterone deficiency. Life will be much simpler for the diagnostic and treating physician if there were, but there isn't.

While it may be a sensible medical practice to routinely measure total testosterone and a range of other factors such as the binding protein in the blood, from which can be calculated the free testosterone, so as to assess at least one of the factors causing hormone resistance, it is not necessary to do it two or three times as often recommended by those keener on denying the patient treatment by taking the lowest values and declaring it to be above an illusory threshold.

Estrogen is seldom measured before HRT is offered to women, so why should there be one rule for women and another for men? If a woman in her forties or fifties has menopausal symptoms and, after discussing the benefits and risks with her doctor, decides to proceed with treatment, that's her choice. Why this sexual discrimination against men with virtually the same symptoms?

Worse still, not only is testosterone treatment often denied to men on the grounds of irrelevant and inaccurate testosterone measurements, but doctors and pharmaceutical companies recommending and selling testosterone preparations are also accused of disease mongering by those who would severely limit the treatment according to blood testosterone levels.[2]

This is disease denial, and failure to offer the treatment to men with the characteristic identikit pattern of symptoms should be treated as a serious failure of medical practice, like failure to recognize and treat diabetes.

It is also dismissed as just a lifestyle drug. If you want to live a long mentally and physically active life, with healthy sexuality, yes, I think most men will say that's a lifestyle they will like.

False Economy

Using any of the above arguments, legislators look around for ways to make savings by cutting back on the drugs bill, especially where a group of doctors can be found to say it is an unnecessary expense.

This happened with Dr Jens Moller in Copenhagen, who was acting as locum for a Dr Tvedegaard, called Dr T for short, when a classic example of trying to economize by limiting the use of testosterone occurred.

Dr. T was often outspoken and critical of his colleagues' attitude and made many enemies among them. More drastic action was needed, and an opportunity for discrediting Dr. Tvedegaard presented itself and was eagerly seized.

In Denmark at that time, the law relating to medicines said that conditions could only be treated with the drugs officially recognized as being effective in those disorders. Because of prevailing medical opinion not only in Denmark but in most other countries as well, testosterone was not on the list of drugs to be used for circulatory problems. Even if an army of a thousand people whose limbs had been saved marched up and down outside the Danish Parliament for a week, the law was the law, and medical opinion could not be moved to change it for sweet reason's sake.

Worse still, patients could have some of the costs of certain vital medicines refunded, provided the condition for which they were given were on the authorized list and the prescriptions were written on the appropriate red forms. Dr. T's deeply held view was that testosterone was a literally life-saving vital medicine, and because it came mainly from the testes, he found a category of genital insufficiency which he thought qualified its use in the cases he saw.

Unfortunately, this came to the notice of the Danish Health Service officials, who reacted in a surprisingly dramatic fashion one day in August 1957. Rather than take the case up through the usual medical disciplinary channels, they sent the state police around the same day to officially charge Dr T and Dr Moller that because testosterone was not a vital medicine, they were betraying the government for money.

This rapidly escalated into a very public cause célèbre with many court hearings, and questions were asked in the Danish Parliament. Dr T's health soon deteriorated under the strain, so Dr Møller, who was made of sterner stuff, was left holding the testosterone baby.

Undeterred by rulings against them in the courts, he mobilized public opinion in their favor. He did a detailed study of the literature and went to Germany to discuss the use of testosterone with the leading endocrinologists of the day, who were very supportive of these ideas. He then organized a public meeting of over fifteen hundred patients and relatives to raise funds for the fight. He lined up doctors from the health authority in the front row, deluged them with this new scientific evidence, and then said, 'Contradict me if you can.' They couldn't and left the hall in a state of confusion and acute embarrassment.

The fight then got very dirty, and the police tried to seize all the patients' case notes and deprive the defendants of their evidence. Dr Møller took the case notes home and piled them in the fireplace, telling his wife to set fire to them if the police called while he was out. The prosecution even made up stories from patients about the way they had been treated, who, when they found out, totally denied them. Fortunately, they had many grateful and influential patients who kept up the legal battle on his behalf as literally, their lives and limbs depended on it.

Eventually, a minister of justice, who was on the State Medical Ethics Committee and had a close relative who was greatly helped by Dr Møller's treatment, got the court's decision reversed and the case called off after a battle which had lasted two years. Not only that, but the director of the Danish Health Authority, who had been one of his fiercest opponents, saw the effects of the treatment on his family and friends and changed to the extent that he became director of LBK, the organization which was set up to promote the use of testosterone.

The facts in this amazing case are documented in a book called *The Tvedegaard Møller Trial: A Fight against Injustice*, written a year later by another Danish doctor who had supported their cause.

Though the medical establishment in Denmark generally remained hostile to the 'Dr Tvedegaard treatment', which they used to tell their students was hormonal humbug, Dr Møller's practice flourished. He used to see fifty or more patients a day, who sometimes had to queue in the street outside his clinic in the fashionable Store Kongensgade (Great King Street), conveniently near his old stamping ground, the Angleterre Hotel, where he was now an honored guest once more.

As was traditional with native prophets, he began receiving much more recognition from the many distinguished doctors from America, Britain, and all over Europe, who came to visit his clinic, than he did from those in Denmark, who seldom came to call except when they wanted research funds from his rapidly growing charitable foundations. Not unnaturally, these experiences left Dr Møller feeling somewhat paranoid, and it became his mission for the rest of his life to hammer home the message of the effectiveness and safety of testosterone.

Another Scandinavian doctor who has been trying to make the case for TRT is Professor Stephan Arver, an endocrine consultant in the Karolinska University in Stockholm, who did an interesting and original cost-benefit analysis of TRT as a preventive medicine. The aim of this analysis was to evaluate health outcomes and costs associated with lifelong TRT in patients suffering from testosterone deficiency.[3]

Using a clever decision program for patients being at continuous risk of disease events called a Markov model, his team assessed the cost-effectiveness of testosterone undecanoate (TU) depot injection treatment compared with no treatment. Health outcomes and associated costs were modeled in monthly cycles per patient individually along a lifetime horizon. Modeled health outcomes included development of type 2 diabetes, depression, cardiovascular and cerebrovascular complications, and fractures.

The main outcome measures were quality-adjusted life years (QALYs) and total cost in TU depot injection treatment and no treatment cohorts. In addition, outcomes were also expressed as incremental cost per QALY gained for TU depot injection therapy compared with no treatment (incremental cost-effectiveness ratio (ICER)).

Outcomes in the testosterone deficient population estimated benefits of TRT at twenty euros (twenty-five USD) per QALY gained. Improvement in the reduced risk of developing type 2 diabetes had the highest impact on long-term outcomes.

This analysis suggests that lifelong TU depot injection therapy of patients with testosterone deficiency is a cost-effective treatment in Sweden and that there is a strong case for doing so, though this has largely been ignored by the authorities. This conclusion is obtained with treatment using injected testosterone and can be even more effective if the cheapest form of treatment with a gel applied to the scrotum, at a third of the cost, has been used.[4]

A similar study in America[5] at Baylor College, Houston, also in 2013, modeled the costs associated with testosterone-related complications, including cardiovascular disease (CVD), diabetes mellitus (DM), and osteoporosis-related fractures (ORFs). Incidence, prevalence, and mortality of these conditions were collected for men aged forty-five to seventy-four from six national databases and large cross-sectional studies. Relative risk (RR) rates were determined for these sequelae in patients with testosterone less than 300 ng/dL (10nmol/L). The prevalence of testosterone deficiency was determined for this cohort of men.

Actual and adjusted (normalized for T deficiency) rates of CVD, DM, and ORFs in US men aged forty-five to seventy-four assuming a TD prevalence of 13.4 percent were calculated. It was determined that, over a twenty-year period, T deficiency is projected to be involved in the development of approximately 1.3 million new cases of CVD, 1.1 million new cases of DM, and over 600,000 ORFs. In year 1, the attributed cost burden of these diseases was approximately $8.4 billion.

It was calculated that over the entire twenty-year period, T deficiency may be directly responsible for approximately $190–$525 billion in inflation-adjusted US health-care expenditures. It was concluded that testosterone deficiency may be a significant contributor to adverse public health and that further study is needed to definitively describe whether testosterone deficiency is a modifiable risk factor for the diseases studied. This may represent an opportunity for nationwide public health initiatives aimed at preventive care.

Despite these carefully quantified financial studies on both sides of the Atlantic on the impact of testosterone deficiency on men's health in financial terms, there still seems remarkably little political will to make testosterone treatment available, even in limited areas, to see what such an experiment in preventive medicine can actually achieve. This may be because politicians are interested in quick fixes rather than immediate expenditure, whose benefits may not be apparent until after the next election in a few years' time. This is known as a limited-event horizon, which dictates much of medical policy.

Medical Insurance Companies and State Providers

Currently, most health insurance companies and state providers in the USA and UK cover neither HRT nor TRT and certainly don't want to do so. However severe the symptoms of the hormonal disturbances which endocrine lack can cause, they regard the resulting conditions as just due to aging, even if they occur midlife and can be reversed by economic hormonal treatments.

They have a strong financial incentive to deny the existence of testosterone deficiency, the treatment costs of which in testosterone products alone, not counting the fees of the doctors administering it and the lab tests, is estimated at 2.2 billion USD annually, though it could and should be made much cheaper.

Certainly, some doctors and medical chains are more profit than medical need orientated, and it is difficult to regulate this, but limiting treatment to patients whose blood test show a low T is definitely not the way. In the process of trying to eliminate patients who do not need treatment, you will deny the large majority who do. History, symptoms, and full clinical assessment, I suggest, are the way forward. It works for HRT; why not TRT?

One troubling development is that several of the pharmaceutical companies marketing testosterone products in the USA using aggressive direct-to-consumer campaigns on television and other media, hyping the dangers of low T, which, as explained previously, is inaccurate in that because of resistance to its action, it is low T activity, which is the problem, have escalated the price of their products to make it an expensive treatment. This is unacceptable to both doctors and the insurance companies as testosterone itself is remarkably cheap to produce from its natural precursor, cholesterol. With it having been available in pure crystalline form for over seventy years, there are little to no development costs, and so there is a very high profit margin.

For example, a month's supply in the UK of one of the most common form of treatment, a gel preparation called Testogel, costs £30. In the USA, it is called AndroGel, comes in a pump dispenser rather than the more economical daily sachets, and costs 310 USD (£210) in the equivalent monthly dosage. This is sort of the markup designed to give testosterone treatment a bad name.

'Aging Naturally' Arguments

There are many opponents of TRT who claim that it is just disease-mongering and choose to ignore the physical and mental benefits of the treatment, which are obvious to those who experience them, to their relatives, and to the doctors prescribing it. If the symptoms go away and stay away on treatment, recur when it is stopped even for a short period, and then go away again when it is resumed, this is not just a placebo effect.

There is a school of thought that adopts an almost moralistic ideology that we should learn to 'grow old gracefully' without medication to improve the quality of later life. This appears to ignore the reality that life expectancy from men has risen from forty-five in 1927 to fifty in 1950 and over eighty in 2000 but that most of this longevity is due to increased periods of frailty and dependency.

For many people, these are not enjoyable or productive years, but miserable and expensive to the individual and society alike. If you get angina and intermittent claudication pain in the legs, have diabetes and suffer from impaired mobility due to a fractured hip, and have to try to live with dementia, these are not desirable ways to grow old gracefully. Without medical intervention in the form of TRT for men and HRT for women, life can become an expensive burden.

Also, particularly in America, there is the religious view that testosterone is all to do with sex, which is mainly for procreation, and is therefore immoral, unseemly, and unnecessary in those over the age of fifty. This ignores the fact that testosterone is not just a sex hormone but has physical functions in relation to body strength and vitality, energy, and enthusiasm.

Many of the same arguments, of course, apply to women, most of whom will like to spend their later life with active, happy, and healthy partners.

Myths of Testosterone Treatment

> The great enemy of truth is very often not the lie—deliberate, contrived and dishonest—but the myth—persistent, persuasive and unrealistic. Too often we hold fast to the clichés of our forebears. We subject all facts to a prefabricated set of interpretations. We enjoy the comfort of opinion without the discomfort of thought.
>
> John F. Kennedy,
> Commencement Address at Yale University,
> 11 June 1962

Nowhere in medicine has the power of myths had a greater influence in holding back progress in the introduction of a medical treatment than in the prominence given to the two great myths about testosterone treatment.

These myths are taught to fledgling medical students, who pass their exams and even get scholarships and awards for reciting them. They constitute fixed ideas in the minds of doctors and medical journalists whenever testosterone treatment is mentioned. Even when comprehensively disproved by the latest medical research, they are trotted out again and again. They resemble the regenerating life of vampires, who have to be nailed to the ground with the crucifix of a definitive rebuttal in a leading journal article. Even then, they are apt to rise again in the minds of older doctors and in articles by less-informed medical and lay journalists who haven't heard, or don't want to know, that the their routinely regurgitated myth has been slain.

Myth Number 1: It May Cause Prostate Cancer

This was the big one that lasted over sixty years, since the idea was dreamt up by a famous American urologist called Charles Huggins. It was based on one patient of his with prostate cancer who appeared to get worse on testosterone replacement treatment (TRT) and temporarily better when treated with the female hormone estrogen, which suppressed release of the hormone.

This simplistic idea became enshrined in the antitestosterone movement, and many prostate cancer victims were physically or chemically castrated to slow the growth of the tumor. This it did for a few months, but at the cost of bringing on the side effects of a testosterone-deficient state, with loss of libido, potency, and brain fog, which often severely reduced his quality of life.

This was seen in the sad closing chapter of a patient I saw at the Middlesex Hospital in London back in the 1960s. Shortly after a successful career as an eminent consultant physician, he developed prostate cancer, and as the urologist treating him worked at the hospital where the synthetic estrogen stilboestrol had been discovered by Sir Charles Dodds in the late 1930s, he was duly put on that drug.

Though it made him feel tired and forgetful, with florid symptoms of chemical testosterone deficiency, he lasted some months with only limited worsening of his prostate cancer, until he went to a family wedding and crashed head-on into another car, several of whose occupants were killed outright. He died depressed about the incident a few months later, a sad ending to an illustrious career.

Also, the idea seemed to ignore the fact that often, it is men with low testosterone levels who develop prostate cancer and that it only becomes common in men over the age of fifty, whose testosterone levels are falling naturally, who develop the condition. Also, intrepid patients using TRT for many years because of the general benefits they have experienced in losing their low-testosterone life and love-limiting symptoms obstinately refuse to develop prostate cancer above the rate experienced by the general population. It was a case of a beautiful theory slain by a few ugly facts. Undeterred, the medical establishment, whenever TRT was mentioned, would appear waving shrouds marked 'Whoa, beware, prostate cancer'.

It was not until a bold young American professor of urology at Harvard Medical School, Abe Morgentaler developed a theory that there was a low threshold of testosterone above which there was no increased risk of cancer.[6]

As he states in the summary of that article, 'studies have failed to show increased risk of PCa in men with higher serum T, and supraphysiologic T fails to increase prostate volume or prostate-specific antigen in healthy men. This apparent paradox is explained by the Saturation Model, which posits a finite capacity of androgen to stimulate PCa growth. Modern studies indicate no increased risk of PCa among men with serum T in the therapeutic range'.

'Fortunately,' Dr. Morgentaler concludes on his highly recommended website, Wellness Profile, and in his excellent, new book, *Testosterone for Life*, 'all of these barriers are now relaxing, as it becomes clear how many body systems rely on healthy, normal T levels, and how normal T levels contribute to prevention of cardiovascular disease, diabetes, and the metabolic syndrome.'

He is even taking his ideas into his clinic, successfully treating some patients who are at high risk of prostate cancer or have had the condition and been treated for it with TRT. This is a complete reversal of the conventional wisdom that TRT is a complete taboo in prostate cancer cases to a situation where it can be judiciously alternated with androgen-deprivation treatment in advanced prostate cancer.[7]

As he states in the summary of this article, 'this prohibition against T therapy has undergone recent re-examination with refinement of our understanding of the biology of androgens and PCa, and increased appreciation of the benefits of T therapy. A reassuringly low rate of negative outcomes has been reported with T therapy after radical prostatectomy (RP), radiation treatments, and in men on active surveillance. Although the number of these published reports are few and the total number of treated men is low, these experiences do provide a basis for consideration of T therapy in selected men with PCa. For clinicians considering offering this treatment, we recommend first selecting patients with low grade cancers and undetectable prostate-specific antigen following RP (Radical Prostatectomey).

'Further research is required to define the safety of T therapy in men with PCa. However, many patients symptomatic from T deficiency are willing to accept the potential risk of PCa progression or recurrence in return for the opportunity to live a fuller and happier life with T therapy'.

His detailed and scholarly attacks on the two main myths of testosterone treatment, that it causes prostate cancer and cardiovascular disease, have surely earned him the title of the 'mighty mythbuster'. The thanks of many patients worldwide and the doctors who treat them are due to him.

His experience coincides with that of consultant urologist Mark Feneley and myself in treating 2,500 patients with TRT over twenty-five years at the Centre for Men's Health, with careful monitoring of the prostate. As reported in the leading *American Journal of Sexual Medicine* in 2012 with an article we dared to call 'Is Testosterone Treatment Good for the Prostate? Study of Safety During Long-Term Treatment',[8] there is no increase in prostate cancer in men having TRT and no rise in the early warning marker, the prostate specific antigen (PSA).

Instead, many men show not only benefits in losing the symptoms of testosterone deficiency but also have improvement in lower urinary tract symptoms, such as frequency of passing water especially at night. This illustrates the point that TRT causes neither benign nor malignant prostate conditions but is good for the health of the entire urinary tract.

Myth Number 2: It May Cause Heart Disease

It seems that doctors enjoy a good myth. Perhaps it makes them seem more knowledgeable and stops them from having to practice a different form of medicine they know little or nothing about.

Just as the prostate cancer myth is in its death throes, a fresh myth is revived to take its place. Those that wish to block the use of TRT have switched their line of reasoning to the mistaken idea that it contributes to cardiovascular disease.[9]

Nowhere is the pull of this second myth put forward more strongly than by advocates of consumer rights. The basic tenet of this movement is that that the consumer, the patient in this case, has the unalienable right to the latest and best treatment without regard to its cost and without any possible side effects.

This view is usually put forward by people outside the medical profession, as those within it tend to have more reasonable expectations. Though believing that treatments and medication should be as safe as possible, they are aware from bitter experience that no treatment is perfectly safe and totally risk free. It is a constant risk–benefit analysis. Even aspirin used to treat your headache can very rarely cause you to bleed to death or have a hemorrhagic stroke which kills you.

In 2014, that bastion of orthodoxy, the *British Medical Journal*, to bolster its largely antitestosterone stance, commissioned an article by the founder and director of a Washington-based organization called Public Citizen entitled 'Increased Heart Attacks in Men Using Testosterone: The UK Importantly Lags far behind the US in Prescribing Testosterone'.[10] For the reasons to be discussed, the first part to this title is questionable, even though the second part is right, but not in the way the authors have intended. Because of restricted prescribing of testosterone in the UK, the US is way ahead in prescribing TRT.

Working initially with consumer rights activist Ralph Nader, Wolfe, seventy-five, and Public Citizen have worked to get twenty-five drugs off the market, pressured the Occupational Safety and Health Administration to set tougher worker health standards, banned Red Dye No. 2, got warning labels about Reye's syndrome on aspirin bottles, and got silicone breast implants restricted, according to the release.

All very worthy causes and a much-needed watchdog over the FDA, especially since its funding was switched from public funding to pharmaceutical company sponsorship. However, this case is based on some dubious recent studies, and if this is the twenty-sixth drug they have taken up cause against, it may be one too far. Undeterred by twenty years of clinical studies showing benefits to the heart and circulation, opponents have based their recent attacks on rising sales figures for testosterone preparations in the US especially and the three flawed studies.

Back in 1945, when TRT was still gaining popularity, an American cardiologist reported that in ten patients, testosterone injections improved angina. Then there was a lull till, during the 1980s, a series of epidemiological articles suggested that low testosterone levels were associated with a greater risk of heart disease and that TRT lowered several risk factors, including blood pressure and cholesterol.

That TRT is beneficial to the heart and circulation was clearly obvious to doctors who use this form of treatment with their patients suffering the classic symptoms of testosterone deficiency syndrome and related disorders. These include diabetes, obesity, metabolic syndrome, osteoporosis, and even Alzheimer's disease. A range of risk factors for heart disease, such as blood pressure, cholesterol, triglycerides, and abdominal obesity, are seen to decrease on the treatment,[11, 12] and especially in diabetics, there is a decrease in heart attack and mortality rates. Then, as seems inevitable with the cyclical nature of research and the varying hemlines of medical research, along comes TOM.

Following twenty years of clinical research showing TRT as being beneficial to the heart, especially in diabetics and in congestive heart failure, an American article alarmingly called 'Association of Testosterone Therapy with Mortality, Myocardial Infarction, and Stroke in Men with Low Testosterone Levels', *The TOM Study: Testosterone in Old Men*, appeared in the prestigious *New England Journal of Medicine* in 2010 and was heavily publicized.

This study, with an impressive list of no fewer than twenty-seven authors from Boston University Endocrinology Department, reports on a study conducted on 209 men sixty-five years or older, half over seventy-five, chosen on the basis of low testosterone levels. These men were not only elderly but also largely immobile, with difficulty even in climbing stairs and walking, but the usual symptoms of testosterone deficiency were not recorded, so we have no way of knowing whether they were really deficient or not other than a very fallible random blood testosterone level.

The researchers then gave these frail, probably confused old men a complicated regime of three packets of testosterone gel or placebo to take, the dose regulated on the basis of blood levels after just two weeks rather than symptom relief, if any. This was likely to result in overdosage in many of the subjects, especially if incorrectly applied. Also, there were more black people in the control group, and they were more prone to overdosage. Baseline readings showed more men with high blood pressure and fat readings in the testosterone-treated group, both risk factors for heart disease.

The article also reported several highly unlikely findings: (1) no increased risk of adverse events up to a body mass index of 40 (morbidly obese), (2) diabetes and smoking halved the rate of adverse events, and (3) high baseline TT halved the risk, while high treatment TT doubled it. The authors themselves concluded, 'The small size of the trial and the unique population prevent broader inferences from being made about the safety of testosterone therapy.' These reservations unfortunately did not however appear in the press reports, and the journalists leapt to draw their own conclusions.

Many experts in testosterone treatment and cardiology agree that this was a thoroughly unsatisfactory study both in design and execution, best summarized as too old, too frail, testosterone too high.

Vigen Study

The second article frequently quoted is by Vigen et al. in *JAMA* in November 2013[13] entitled 'Association of Testosterone Therapy with Mortality, Myocardial Infarction, and Stroke in Men With Low Testosterone Levels'.

It economized in only having twelve authors but made up for it in being based on a vast retrospective study of 8,709 men from the Veterans Affairs system who were having coronary angiography between 2005 and 2011. The problem of such large groups is that there is very little data on each patient available for detailed assessment and that factors which are not clinically or biologically significant can be made statistically significant.

The approach of the authors is given in the summary in that the stated importance of the article as given in the abstract was that it agreed with the concerns raised by the few previous adverse reports, not that it disagreed with most of the clinical studies over the previous twenty years.

To start with, it was unlikely that those having any sort of testosterone for even the briefest period had adequate or properly administered treatment. The testosterone started, on average, eighteen months after angiography and only lasted up to the cutoff point at three years, suggesting that half the time, patients in the treatment group were not on testosterone.

When they were, only 13 (1.1 percent) had what might be considered adequate and consistent treatment, testosterone gel. Of the 8,709 men with a total testosterone level lower than 300 ng/dL, 1,223 patients started testosterone therapy after a median of 531 days following coronary angiography. Of the 1,710 outcome events in this group of men at high risk of vascular disease, overall, 748 men died (8.5 percent), 443 had MIs (5.1 percent), and 519 (6.0 percent) had strokes. Of 7,486 patients not receiving testosterone therapy, 681 died (9.1 percent), 420 had MIs (5.6 percent), and 486 (6.5 percent) had strokes. Among 1,223 patients receiving testosterone therapy, 67 died (5.5 percent), 23 had MIs (1.9 percent), and 33 (2.7 percent) had strokes, simple statistics suggesting a clear benefit to the testosterone-treated group. These findings were reversed by the use of sophisticated statistics using stabilized inverse probability of weighting techniques and used to show the alleged dangers of TRT to the heart. This conforms to the old saying that if you torture statistics long enough, they will confess to anything.

The few adequately treated gel-treated patients were facing heroic odds when set against approximately 2.9 percent of men over the age of forty on TRT in the USA (nearly one and a half million) currently using the medication with sufficient benefit to wish to continue and without clinically obvious adverse side effects.

Expert clinicians in the field worldwide were left speechless and wrote letters of protest to the editor of *JAMA* and other journals and raged at conferences about the design of the study and the statistical analyses used. Where is the balance of evidence on which to issue such alarmist health warnings?

In summary, this study could be summarized as a study with too many patients and dubious statistical techniques used to reverse the initial findings.

The publicity over this article had an immediate adverse effect on the public image of TRT, which is continuing to this day. If you look up Google trends under interest in 'low testosterone' on the web you will see that before these articles in 2013 there was a peak of around 100 hits per day which fell to 53 by the end of 2015. Many US physicians in the TRT field report a continuing halving of patients going on and staying on treatment. This echoes the lasting damage to the health of women on HRT caused by the now largely discredited Women's Health Initiative (WHI) study.

The myths surrounding these important and effective means of preventive medicine and treatment are having a deadly effect on their use.

PLOS ONE Study

Thirdly, a paper in a relatively seldom quoted and low-ranking, open-access journal, PloS One, was published in January 2014 entitled 'Increased Risk of Non-Fatal Myocardial Infarction Following Testosterone Therapy Prescription in Men'.[14] Following the other two studies and quoting them as reasons for the one, the mainly commercial statistician authors used insurance data on 55,593 men who filled a first prescription for any of several testosterone prescriptions. These included testosterone gel, micronized testosterone cypionate injections, and testosterone patches. Again, the numbers are so great that the clinically insignificant factors become statistically significant.

The main potential weakness of this trial is the control group of 167,279 men who took PDE5 inhibitors. This leads to confusion in the selection of a group who may have silent coronary disease and who are therefore completely unsuitable as a control group. Men who are known to have heart disease, especially those with angina, and on coronary vasodilator drugs are not supposed to take these drugs and would have been excluded by their physicians. These considerations alone should have invalidated the study and prevented it from being published.

Misled by studies such as the three above and their unjustified conclusions, the orthodox medical establishment and the general public are being unduly alarmed about the possibility of an association between testosterone treatment and circulatory disease.

Attempting to Trash the Case for Testosterone Treatment

This has long been a favorite technique for opponents of the treatment, especially when losing the scientific case. The most common approach is to use the following ten golden rules for trying to demolish the case for testosterone treatment:

1. *Start by invoking commercial greed and disease-mongering on the part of Big Pharma* as the cause of the large increase in testosterone prescriptions in North America. Produce alarming statistics about US pharmaceutical sales of testosterone increasing from $324 million in 2002 to $2billion in 2012, and the number of testosterone prescriptions climbing from 100 million in 2002 to half a billion in 2012.

   Impressive figures certainly, but how much of this increase is due to the effectiveness of direct-to-consumer product advertising (DTCPA) and how much to increased public awareness of the causes and symptoms of testosterone deficiency and increasing demand for the relief of these symptoms and associated conditions, such as osteoporosis and diabetes? This is combined with a reduced fear of prostate cancer among prescribers.

As has been pointed out by Prof. Abe Morgentaler in 2010 during the steepest increase in testosterone prescriptions, no testosterone product is within the top-twenty most-advertised drugs. This suggests that DTCPA is only a partial explanation at best and a fat red herring at worst.

2. *Set your own standards for the diagnosis of late-onset hypogonadism and ignore any evidence to the contrary.* Insist on the purely laboratory diagnosis of the condition based on low testosterone levels, regardless of the fallacies involved in doing so, and the lack of relationship of these with clinical symptoms and conditions or prognosis on treatment.

3. *Play up the myths* of dangers, such as prostate cancer and cardiovascular disease, even if these fears have been disproved. Ignoring thirty years' worth of evidence to the contrary, insist that there is no convincing evidence that testosterone treatment of age-related hypogonadism is safe.

4. *Associate the testosterone treatment* with other drugs of unproven benefit, such as growth hormone.

5. *Link TRT with the fallacious findings in relation to HRT arising from the Women's Health Initiative (WHI)* study even if the findings of that one product study has largely been disproved.

6. *Associate testosterone deficiency purely with aging* and maintain that treating it is therefore unjustified and meddling with nature. While choosing your own terms carefully, remember at all times that by definition, *Age-related hypogonadism* is a rare condition diagnosed on the basis of an assumed normal distribution of testosterone at different ages of 0.5 percent[15] rather than the 40 percent of the over forty-fives suggested by some authors[16] who take more account of symptoms.

7. *March under the banner of science-based medicine* even if it is in fact opinion based and this basis crumbles under closer scrutiny.

8. *Dismiss all opponents of your views* as disease-mongering permissive prescribers using lax, distorted clinical judgment. The terms *quackery* and *huxterism* are useful here. In other words, deride all those practicing outside the true faith of so-called modern scientific medicine however fallible and incomplete that science may be. Whatever the results they get and however satisfied their patients are, they are heretics.

9. *Join with others* who have similar views to your own and form a chorus of opposition.

10. *Air your views loudly* and repetitively at conferences and in journal articles, obeying Lewis Carroll's dictum in the hunting of the Snark, 'What I tell you three times is true' however apparently nonsensical it proves when carefully analyzed.

To show how worthless these ten golden rules are, I suggest you consider the following logic.

Testosterone levels are largely invalid as measures of testosterone deficiency[17] because of the following:

1. *Preanalytical factors* (The exact sampling conditions in relation to circadian and seasonal variations, diet, alcohol, physical activity, and posture.)

2. *Physiological and medical factors* (Androgen levels vary according to the patient's biological age, his physical and mental health, stress, sexual activity, and smoking habits.)

3. *Analytical variables* (Sample preservation and storage are often unknown, different androgen assays have widely different accuracy and precision and are subject to large interlaboratory variation exhortations to use GCMS, and take multiple samples that are expensive and often impractical in routine clinical practice.)

4. *Interpretation of results* (Laboratory reference ranges vary widely, largely independent of methodology, and fail to take into account the log-normal distribution of androgen values, all causing errors in clinical diagnosis and treatment.)

5. *Internal androgen resistance*[18] (Impaired androgen synthesis or regulation, increased androgen binding, reduced tissue responsiveness, decreased androgen receptor activity, impaired transcription and translation.)

There is no relationship between testosterone levels and symptoms, associated conditions, and the response to testosterone treatment.[19] This is hardly surprising in view of the first two factors but is totally ignored by those bent on denying testosterone treatment to patients.

Consequences of Testosterone Resistance

The reality of testosterone resistance is that it is a game changer; it changes the thinking about the causes, diagnosis, and treatment of testosterone deficiency.

References for Chapter 4

1. M. Carruthers, T. R. Trinick, and M. J. Wheeler, 'The Validity of Androgen Assays', *CPD Clinical Biochemistry*, 8/3 (2007), 82–89.

2. D. J. Handelsman, 'Pharmacoepidemiology of testosterone prescribing in Australia, 1992–2010', *Medical Journal of Australia*, 196/10 (2012), 642–645.

3. S. Arver, B. Luong, A. Fraschke, O. Ghatnekar, S. Stanisic, D. Gultyev, et al., 'Is Testosterone Replacement Therapy in Males with Hypogonadism Cost-Effective? An Analysis in Sweden', *Journal of Sexual Medicine* (2013).

4. M. Carruthers, P. J. Cathcart, and M. R. Feneley, 'Evolution of Testosterone Treatment over 25 Years: Symptom Responses, Endocrine Profiles and Cardiovascular Changes', *The Aging Male* (2015).

5. D. J. Moskovic, A. B. Araujo, L. I. Lipshultz, and M. Khera, 'The 20-Year Public Health Impact and Direct Cost of Testosterone Deficiency in US Men', *The Journal of Sexual Medicine*, 10/2 (2013), 562–569.

6. A. Morgentaler, 'Testosterone and Prostate Cancer: What Are the Risks for Middle-Aged Men?', *Urologic Clinics of North America*, 38/2 (2011), 119–124.

7. A. Morgentaler and W. P. Conners III, 'Testosterone Therapy in Men with Prostate Cancer: Literature Review, Clinical Experience, and Recommendations', *Asian Journal of Andrology*, 17/2 (2015), 206–211.

8. M. R. Feneley and M. Carruthers, 'Is Testosterone Treatment Good for the Prostate? Study of Safety during Long-Term Treatment', *Journal of Sexual Medicine*, 9 (2012), 2,138–2,149.

9. S. M. Wolfe, 'Increased Heart Attacks in Men Using Testosterone: The UK Importantly Lags Far behind the US in Prescribing Testosterone', *The BMJ*, 348 (2014), g1789.

10. Ibid.

11. R. Stanworth and T. Jones, 'Testosterone in Obesity, Metabolic Syndrome and Type 2 Diabetes', *Frontiers of Hormone Research*, 37 (2009), 74–90.

12. T. H. Jones, S. Arver, H. M. Behre, J. Buvat, E. Meuleman, I. Moncada, et al., 'Testosterone Replacement in Hypogonadal Men with Type 2 Diabetes and/or Metabolic Syndrome (The TIMES2 study)', *Diabetes Care*, 34/4 (2011), 828–837.

13. R. Vigen, C. I. O'Donnell, A. E. Barón, G. K. Grunwald, T. M. Maddox, S. M. Bradley, et al., 'Association of Testosterone Therapy with Mortality, Myocardial Infarction, and Stroke in Men with Low Testosterone Levels', *Journal of the American Medical Association*, 310/17 (2013), 1,829–1,836.

14. W. D. Finkle, S. Greenland, G. K. Ridgeway, J. L. Adams, M. A. Frasco, M. B. Cook, et al., 'Increased Risk of Non-Fatal Myocardial Infarction Following Testosterone Therapy Prescription in Men', *PLoS ONE*, 9/1 (2014), e85805.

15. F. C. Wu, A. Tajar, J. M. Beynon, S. R. Pye, A. J. Silman, J. D. Finn, et al., 'Identification of Late-Onset Hypogonadism in Middle-Aged and Elderly Men', *New England Journal of Medicine*, 362 (2010), 1–13.

[16.] T. Mulligan, M. F. Frick, Q. C. Zuraw, A. Stemhagen, and C. McWhirter, 'Prevalence of Hypogonadism in Males Aged at Least 45 Years: The HIM Study', *International Journal of Clinical Practice*, 60/7 (2006), 762–769.

[17.] Carruthers M, Trinick TR, Wheeler MJ. The validity of androgen assays. *Aging Male* 2007; 10(3):165-172.

[18.] M. Carruthers, 'The Paradox Dividing Testosterone Deficiency Symptoms and Androgen Assays: A Closer Look at the Cellular and Molecular Mechanisms of Androgen Action', *Journal of Sexual Medicine*, 5/4 (2008) 998–1,012.

[19.] M. Carruthers, P. J. Cathcart, and M. R. Feneley, 'Evolution of Testosterone Treatment over 25 Years: Symptom Responses, Endocrine Profiles and Cardiovascular Changes', *The Aging Male* (2015).

Chapter 5
What Testosterone Resistance Means in Terms of Diagnosis

There are two ways to be fooled. One is to believe what isn't true;
the other is to refuse to believe what is true.
Søren Kierkegaard, Danish Philosopher, 1813-1855

Most of the opponents of testosterone treatment cleverly manage to make both errors at the same time.

This new idea of testosterone resistance means going back to the drawing board for both the diagnosis and treatment of testosterone deficiency.

Once you have accepted the principle, the evidence for its existence and importance falls into place.

Firstly, the idea that blood tests are the gold standard for deciding whether a man is deficient falls by the wayside. When you examine the sampling problems, the laboratory measurement problems, and the interpretation problems, you realize that from being the measure of the condition, it is fool's gold. It is not low T, as the adverts say, but low T activity, a very different thing.

So out go all the ideas of screening campaigns for finding low testosterone levels in the community in favor of making men aware of the symptoms of testosterone deficiency and helping them recognize the key features. They should seek help if and when they need it or develop a related condition such as diabetes. You won't suggest screening for the menopause in women, will you?

By all means, measure the testosterone levels once the diagnosis has been established on a symptomatic basis, preferably using Prof. Lothar Heineman's excellent aging male symptoms (AMS) questionnaire.[1] This is available free in twenty languages, has been fully validated, and is also available online (www.andropause. org.uk). This simple but effective diagnostic tool is also given in full, together with the scoring system, at the end of this book. The seventeen questions are each rated 1–5, and a total score of over 37 makes the diagnosis of testosterone deficiency moderately likely, and over 50 highly probable.

When the AMS questionnaire was completed in a web survey by over 10,000 men, mainly from the UK and USA, of who responded, 80 percent had moderate or severe scores, likely to benefit from TRT.[2] The average age of these men was fifty-two, many cases in their forties, an age when the diagnosis of late-onset hypogonadism is not generally considered. Other possible contributory factors to the high testosterone deficiency scores reported were obesity (29 percent), alcohol (17.3 percent), testicular problems such as mumps orchitis (11.4 percent), prostate problems (5.6 percent), urinary infection (5.2 percent), and diabetes (5.7 percent) (figure 1).

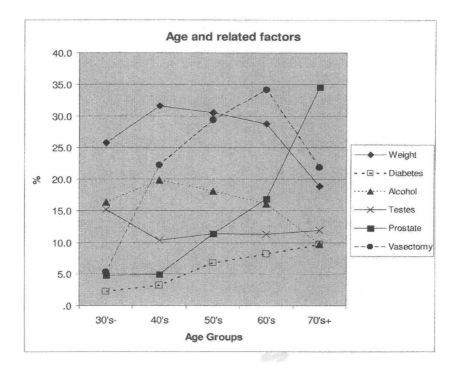

Figure 1. Additional factors reported in the different age groups

It was concluded that in this self-selected large international sample of men, there was a very high prevalence of scores which would warrant a therapeutic trial of testosterone treatment. The study suggested that there are large numbers of men in the community whose testosterone deficiency was neither being diagnosed nor treated.

The lack of relationship between blood testosterone levels and the symptoms has been clearly shown in the UK Androgen Study of men presenting for TRT with symptoms of deficiency over the last twenty-five years[3] to establish the symptom response when testosterone treatment was initiated on the basis of clinical features and symptoms of androgen deficiency and the resulting endocrine, biochemical, and physiological responses.

Of 2,693 patients attending the three Men's Health Centres (The UK Androgen Study (UKAS)), 2,247 were treated. Treatments included pellet implants, oral testosterone undecanoate (Testocaps), mesterolone (Proviron), testosterone gel (Testogel), testosterone scrotal cream (Andromen), and scrotal gel (Tostran).

There was no correlation between initial testosterone level, initial symptom score, or the success of treatment as defined by adequate resolution of symptoms. Despite the diverse endocrine patterns produced, the testosterone preparations appear equally safe over prolonged periods, with either no change or improvement of cardiovascular risk factors, especially in lowering cholesterol and diastolic blood pressure.

However, the initial findings clearly showed that there was no significant increase in total symptom scores over the full range of total and free testosterone (figure 2).

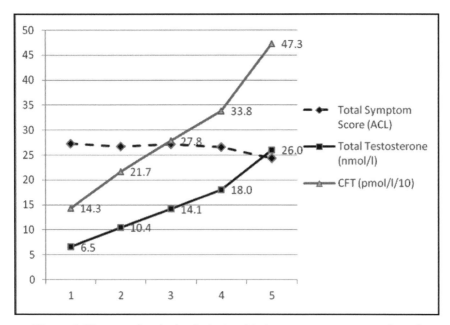

Figure 2. The complete lack of relationship between symptoms and total testosterone or calculated free testosterone (CFT) at the first visit

Also, the initial level of testosterone was no use in assessing whether the patient would respond to treatment or not (figure 3). Those who started on treatment with symptoms and a high total testosterone responded just as well as those that might have been diagnosed on the basis of their low total testosterone. In other words, total testosterone is of no use in diagnosis or prognosis.

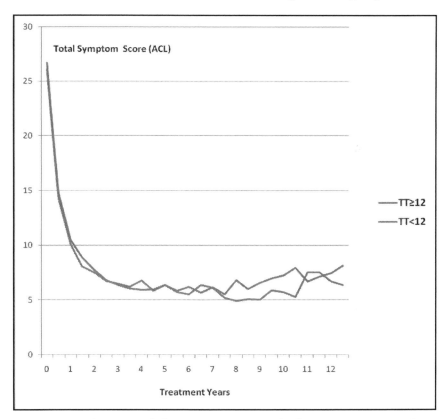

Figure 3. There is no difference in symptom relief between patients with initial testosterone levels above and below the commonly accepted cutoff point of 12 nmol/L.

Other researchers have confirmed the way that testosterone levels are not related to symptoms, but still they are used as the basis of the diagnosis of testosterone deficiency. Take for example these quotations from the summaries of their articles:

1. 'There was no correlation between AMS (total and subscales) and testosterone levels.'[4]

2. 'None of the three AMS domain scale scores significantly correlated with testosterone, free testosterone or bioavailable testosterone. Significant correlations were observed between results for the AMS scores and those for other health questionnaires, but none of the subscores for the latter questionnaires correlated with androgen serum levels.'[5]

3. 'None of the three AMS domain scale scores and total scores significantly correlated with serum levels of TT, FT, E2, LH, FSH, DHEA-S, or GH.'[6]

4. 'The lack of correlation between the clinical picture and the most commonly used biochemical confirmatory tests (TT, SHBG, LH), again, clearly points to the paramount importance of the clinical evaluation. An emphasis and reliance on serum T alone hinders the clinician's ability to manage testosterone deficiency syndromes (TDS).'[7]

5. A problem with the diagnosis of LOH is that often the symptoms (in 20%-40% of unselected men) and low circulating T (in 20% of men >70 years of age) do not coincide in the same individual.' By combining these criteria 'only 2% of 40- to 80-year-old men have LOH.'[8]

Nice one, this, though the logic is unclear. Why, if the two diagnostic tests for a condition don't agree, then insist on using both of them together.

6. 'The search for a discrete threshold may be futile given emerging evidence. Recent studies suggest that testosterone threshold varies by symptoms and among individuals. In addition, thresholds may vary between young and old men. Therefore, initiation of treatment should rely more on symptoms and less on a discrete numerical threshold.'[9]

Diagnosing according mainly to blood testosterone levels as measured before treatment is also guaranteed to miss a large proportion of cases of testosterone deficiency.

The likely percentage of symptomatic cases receiving treatment is shown in figure 4 and varies from 2 percent, if the latest ruling of Australian Pharmaceutical Benefits Committee, which puts the threshold of total testosterone at 6 nmol/L, to a generous 17 percent, if the level of 12 nmol/L put forward by the majority of European agencies is observed. Not until the level of about 27 nmol/L is reached are all symptomatic cases included as being eligible for treatment.

Looked at another way, what clinician would decide his clinical practice on the basis of a test which appears to have a false-negative rate of over 80 percent?

There is no Threshold
- TT no use in diagnosis

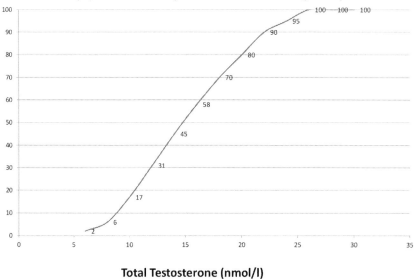

Figure 4. Percentage of patients who obtained remission of symptoms in the UK Androgen Study according to their initial testosterone levels.

References for Chapter 5

1. L. A. J. Heinemann, T. Zimmermann, A. Vermeulen, C. Thiel, and W. Hummel, 'A New "Aging Males' Symptoms" (AMS) Rating Scale', The Aging Male, 2/2 (1999), 105–114.

2. T. R. Trinick, M. R. Feneley, H. Welford, and M. Carruthers, 'International Web Survey Shows High Prevalence of Symptomatic Testosterone Deficiency in Men', The Aging Male, 14/1 (2011), 10–15.

3. M. Carruthers, P. J. Cathcart, and M. R. Feneley, 'Evolution of Testosterone Treatment over 25 Years: Symptom Responses, Endocrine Profiles and Cardiovascular Changes', The Aging Male (2015).

4. G. T'Sjoen, E. Feyen, P. De Kuyper, F. Comhaire, and J. M. Kaufman, 'Self-Referred Patients in an Aging Male Clinic: Much More Than Androgen Deficiency Alone', The Aging Male, 6/3 (2003), 157–165.

5. G. T'Sjoen, S. Goemaere, M. De Meyere, and J. M. Kaufman, 'Perception of Males' Aging Symptoms, Health and Well-Being in Elderly Community-Dwelling Men Is Not Related to Circulating Androgen Levels', Psychoneuroendocrinology, 29/2 (2004), 201–214.

6. Y. Miwa, T. Kaneda, and O. Yokoyama, 'Correlation between the Aging Males' Symptoms Scale and Sex Steroids, Gonadotropins, Dehydroepiandrosterone Sulfate, and Growth Hormone Levels in Ambulatory Men', Journal of Sexual Medicine, 3/4 (2006), 723–726.

7. A. Morales, M. Spevack, L. Emerson, I. Kuzmarov, R. Casey, A. Black, et al., 'Adding to the Controversy: Pitfalls in the Diagnosis

of Testosterone Deficiency Syndromes with Questionnaires and Biochemistry', The Aging Male, 10/2 (2007), 57–65.

[8.] I. Huhtaniemi, 'Late-Onset Hypogonadism: Current Concepts and Controversies of Pathogenesis, diagnosis and Treatment', Asian Journal of Andrology, 16 (2014), 192–202.

[9.] A. Maganty, J. E. Shoag, and R. Ramasamy, 'Testosterone Threshold: Does One Size Fit All?', *The Aging Male* (2015), 1–4.

Chapter 6
Treating Testosterone Deficiency

The idea of testosterone resistance profoundly alters the approach to both diagnosis and treatment. In treating a man with symptoms of testosterone deficiency or a related condition such as diabetes, you not only have to raise the testosterone level but also consider ways of reducing resistance to its action. As in diabetes, you are treating either an absolute or relative deficiency of a hormone.

Testing for Testosterone Resistance

Firstly, though you don't need to do it routinely, you can test for testosterone resistance. You can suspect it in most cases, certainly below the age of fifty, by the high level of testosterone in the presence of clear symptoms. Where this is not the case, you can confirm the resistance by a therapeutic trial of an injection of a long-acting preparation, such as testosterone undecanoate (Nebido in the UK and Europe (1 g), Reandron in Australia (1 g), or Aveed in the USA (0.75 g)).

The 1 g injections are designed to last up to three months, where there is low resistance as in young men with primary testicular failure, nondescent, or orchidectomy for testicular cancer. Too often, urological surgeons removing one testis pat their young patients on the back and say, 'You still have the other testis. You'll be fine.' But within two or three years, they develop symptoms of testosterone deficiency, which are frequently not recognized or are ignored rather than relieved by TRT as part of the routine follow-up.

However, the typical patient in their fifties notice that their symptoms improve for a shorter time after the 1 g injection, say, six weeks, so that what could be called the testosterone resistance index (TRI) is 12/6, i.e. 2, rather than 12/12, i.e. 1. This is where the resistance is often due to multiple causes such as age, stress, alcohol, medications, or diabetes.

This test is simple to carry out and, if positive, can be followed by whatever treatment the clinician finds most effective. It can be compared to the glucose tolerance test for diabetics.

Testosterone Replacement Therapy (TRT)

The choice of testosterone treatment is much wider than it has been twenty-five years ago, as considered in my article on 'The Evolution of Testosterone Treatment',[1] with more options in the UK and Australia than in the USA.

Each of the seven different form of testosterone treatment used over the previous twenty-five years can prove clinically effective when the patients are selected on the basis of the diagnostic symptoms, and to paraphrase the saying from George Orwell's *Animal Farm*, all treatments are equal, but some are more equal than others. It depends largely on the degree of resistance, costs of maintaining the treatment, and the patient's and clinician's preferences.

Treatments include pellet implants, oral testosterone undecanoate (Testocaps), mesterolone (Proviron), testosterone gel (Testogel), testosterone undecanoate injections (Nebido), testosterone scrotal cream (Andromen), and scrotal gel (Tostran). With the exception of mesterolone, which only has a weak therapeutic action, all treatments appear effective and safe, but the scrotal preparations have considerable price advantages.

Reducing the Resistance to Testosterone

Raising testosterone levels to overcome the resistance has been the mainstay of treatment since testosterone became available over seventy years ago. However, this does not overcome the root cause, may reduce the body's natural testosterone production, and needs to be maintained lifelong. Many of the measures needed to do so come under the heading of lifestyle modification, seldom an easy thing to achieve.

However, TRT creates a window of opportunity by boosting willpower and 'won't power', that he will reduce his intake of sugar and starches and won't snack, that he will take more exercise and become less of a couch potato. Results can be slow, but over a one year, studies have shown that patients can develop improved musculature and lose weight.[2]

Weight Reduction

It's the old 'calories in, calories out' equation. Reducing and decreasing the portion and size and switching away from sugar and carbohydrate toward protein and vegetable oils are the bases. The Atkins diet series of books are very good for helping this process and are thoroughly recommended. Another effectives so-called '5:2 diet' (5 days normal and 2days fasting) is described in a recent book by the English writer Dr Michael Moseley. A dietary pact with your partner can be very helpful here.

Alcohol is a key source of calories and can sap morale as well as generate stress. Beer also contains xenoestrogens and can cause weight gain.

Exercise should be gentle and progressive, vigorous but not violent, and dynamic rather than static. Walking for ten, fifteen, twenty minutes per day is a good start and can reduce stress levels, especially if undertaken with a dog. Cycling and rowing on a rowing machine are also suitable, noncompetitive forms of exercise for those over fifty.

Swimming is a particularly good form of exercise. You can be said to get double-bubble benefit with swimming. It is the right type of whole-body exercise, and you are burning off extra calories even in comfortably warm water.

A personal exercise trainer can be a good investment if you can afford it.

Stress Reduction

As well as directly reducing testosterone production, stress creates testosterone resistance by causing the release of the stress hormones epinephrine (adrenaline), norepinephrine (noradrenaline), cortisol, and a pituitary gland hormone called prolactin.

Rather than relying on drugs to reduce stress, stress-reduction methods should be employed within the limits of your lifestyle—not becoming a stress-avoiding vegetable but becoming aware of the performance-arousal curve.

This views stress as a force like electricity in your life. A certain amount is necessary to stimulate you and help you perform at your optimal level. It's when you go into overload that it can cause you to blow a fuse and burn out. You need to know and accept whether you are a thirty-amp-cooker-fuse type of person or a possibly more creative three-amp-lighting-fuse sort of person (figure 1).

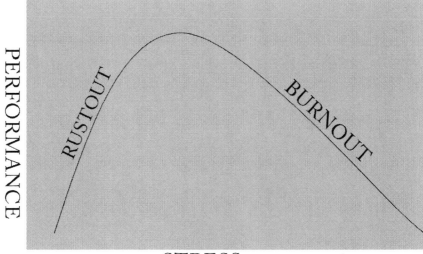

Figure 1. Performance-stress curve

Adequate sleep, which is the time when most testosterone is secreted, is essential to help you resist stress. This needs to be naturally obtained and not with the help of sleeping pills. This requires a regime of sleep-hygiene, involving a regular bedtime, no caffeinated drinks after 6:00 p.m., only one or two alcoholic drinks generally per evening, and switching off your exposure to computers and violent, worrying TV programs and films late at night. Sorry, but your brain needs to wind its activity down an hour or so before you go to sleep.

The many-millennia-old solution to stress through meditation is an ideal antidote to stress and is becoming very popular both in the UK and US. This involves sitting in a quiet place and simply turning one's attention within. You don't have to change your religion as many forms are nonsectarian. Christian prayer, Buddhist and Hindu mantra meditations, and even breath-watching, mindful meditation can all prove very relaxing and improve your experience of life. Meditation, not medication, should be your aim.

My personal choice is Siddha meditation (perfect meditation), an ancient nonsectarian form which is taught free of charge at over 300 centers worldwide.

References for Chapter 6

[1] M. Carruthers, P. J. Cathcart, and M. R. Feneley MR, 'Evolution of Testosterone Treatment over 25 Years: Symptom Responses, Endocrine Profiles and Cardiovascular Changes', *The Aging Male* (2015).

[2] A. Yassin, D. J. Yassin, A. Traish, G. Doros, and F. Saad, 'Long-Term Testosterone Treatment Leads to Progressive Weight Loss and Waist Size Reduction in Hypogonadal Men', *Journal of Urology*, 191/4 (2014).

Chapter 7
Fighting Testosterone Resistance in the World

'Are you planning to follow a career in Magical Laws, Miss Granger?' asked Scrimgeour. 'No, I'm not,' retorted Hermione. 'I'm hoping to do some good in the world!'

J. K. Rowling

quoted by Siddhartha Mukherjee

in his book *The Laws of Medicine*

In this final chapter we will see how at present, the established 'magical laws' of medicine are winning hands down over the natural desire of the doctor to do some good in the world.

Mukherjee puts forward three very practical new laws which seem to apply to the theme of this book, *Testosterone Resistance.* We will take each in turn.

Law 1: A Strong Intuition Is Much More Powerful than a Weak Test

Certainly, in the diagnosis of testosterone deficiency, the doctor's overall assessment, combined with his detailed, standardized questionnaire, is far better than the currently favored total testosterone measured in the blood or any other lab test come to that.

The total testosterone well fits the definition of a weak test as it is inaccurate[1] and misleading, missing up to 90 percent of cases that can benefit from treatment,[2] and denies treatment to millions of men worldwide with the indentikit symptoms of testosterone deficiency.

Law 2: 'Normals' Teach Us Rules, Outliers Teach Us Laws

Based on lab tests, usually total testosterone, most doctors try and achieve a procrustean fit for the patient within the so-miscalled normal range of lab values. Outliers on this scale teach us the law that you can have rampant and health-threatening symptoms of testosterone deficiency yet have high levels of testosterone.

Like the high levels of insulin in some diabetic patients, a high level of testosterone well up or even above the so-called normal range can coexist with severe symptoms of deficiency which are rapidly cured by giving TRT, teaching us the law of testosterone resistance.

Also, when a young man in his thirties with advanced disease of the arteries of both legs, which has failed to respond to extensive surgery and where amputation appears the only answer, responds dramatically to TRT, ignore him. He is an outlier. When he is skiing and teaching tai chi on both legs twenty-five years later, still on high-dose TRT, he can safely be ignored as an outlier and, worst still, an embarrassment to his surgeons, who have made the diagnosis of hopeless progressive arterial disease and advised amputation.

Law 3: For Every Perfect Medical Experiment There Is a Perfect Human Bias

This certainly applies to research into testosterone treatment, where for every one of the thousands of encouraging trials showing the positive effects of TRT in relief of symptoms, coronary heart disease, osteoporosis, frailty, and debility, you can find a few negative ones. These are usually based on opinion rather than fact, which will criticize, deny, or oppose it. We have looked at the many of the sources of this bias against TRT in this book.

As a result of the application and distortion of the 'magical laws' conjured up by modern superscientific medicine, I frankly think we are going in reverse as far as the availability of testosterone treatment is concerned both in the UK and in the US and, worst of all, in Australia.

This is similar to the turning of the tide of medical and, consequently, public opinion against HRT by two highly publicized studies which were published early this century and, looking back, appeared designed to create a climate of fear. The first was the Women's Health Initiative. Started in 1991 by the National Institute of Health in the USA, it was the largest and most expensive clinical research ever conducted into women's health, involving over 16,000 women, mainly in their sixties and seventies, who had an intact uterus and another 10,000 hystectomized group. The first received Premarin (equine estrogen), though had long been regarded as the least-favorable form of HRT, plus Provera (medroxyprogesterone acetate); these were at least cheap and made a huge study possible. The second group received Provera only or a placebo.

One interesting fact about equine estrogen which was known even before the WHI study started was that unlike other natural estrogens, it actually reduced the amount of free estrogens and testosterone in the blood by increasing the binding protein hormone-binding globulin. But that unintended consequence didn't stop the wrong preparations from being used.

When it was time to publish the results, unfortunately, the writing group, in what has since been described as an extraordinary decision in a recently published book *Managing the Menopause*, released their results to health reporters on 10 July, one week prior to the publication of the evidence in *JAMA*. This tactic appeared designed to induce maximum fear and confusion before the general medical profession had a chance to review the evidence.

Also, it seemed that the results had been deliberately reported in relative values rather than absolute values as a deliberate attempt to magnify the adverse events and strike fear into the minds of women and their clinicians using HRT. In this it succeeded brilliantly, and majority of women on HRT worldwide came off it on what, when properly analyzed, was insufficient evidence.

The long-term finding was that after eleven years and much misery from withdrawal, the risk of stroke was not increased, the risk of deep vein thrombosis was decreased, and the risk of breast cancer was reduced by 23 percent. Also, the risk of hip fracture was increased by 55 percent when a woman stopped her HRT, but still, many doctors turned their minds and opinions against HRT, choosing the do-nothing option, and strongly advised against it. Neither was the marriage-breakdown rate recorded in the untreated group. What an expensive public health disaster! Yet still, the misreported findings of the WHI study were also routinely used as evidence against any enthusiasm expressed for TRT.

The second was the Million Women Study which appeared in 2003 in that bastion of orthodoxy, *The Lancet*. Not only did the study make no allowance for women changing from their original form of HRT, but a review in 2011 also reported that the findings did not satisfy the criteria of time order, information bias, cofounding, statistical stability and strength of association, duration response, internal consistency, external consistency, or biological plausibility. The criticism seemed damning, but the damage to HRT had been done.

Typical of this hardening of the forces resistant to the use of testosterone for the treatment of what they will insist terming *age-related hypogonadism* is the latest pronouncement of the Federal Drug Administration (FDA)[3] in that bastion of orthodoxy, the *New England Journal of Medicine*. After reiterating the causes of relatively rare classic hypogonadism with obvious testicular malfunction, the authors make the interesting statement that the FDA only require that testosterone products 'reliably bring low serum concentrations into the normal range for healthy young men.'

This makes two fundamental erroneous assumptions within the first paragraph of the article. Firstly is that the condition can be defined in terms of testosterone levels at any age regardless of testosterone resistance and, secondly, that the aim of treatment is to bring serum concentrations to within the normal range for young men, whatever that may be. The aim of treatment for most practicing clinicians is not to achieve any particular arbitrary level of testosterone but to alleviate the patient's symptoms or associated conditions.

What they go on to describe is the controversial condition that the FDA calls age-related or late-onset hypogonadism, even if it occurs in men in their forties, which may cause men over that age, expecting to live twice as long, to object. Then comes the traditional charge that in these cases, it is unclear (for which read we don't believe) 'whether co-existing nonspecific signs and symptoms, such as decreases in energy and muscle mass, are a consequence of the age-related decline in endogenous testosterone or whether they are a result of other factors, such as coexisting conditions, concomitant medications, or perhaps aging itself'.

For the many reasons already given, it is not the highly characteristic symptoms, which are nonspecific, but the unrelated and highly fallible blood testosterone levels, which, except in extreme cases, are nonspecific.

Following the traditional plea that not enough is known about the risks of TRT and a brief review of the conflicting studies on whether or not there may be increased risk of cardiovascular disease, big advisory organizations—which they usually do when they want to delay making a decision—in September 2014 convened an advisory committee, saying that 'the available evidence supports an indication for testosterone therapy only in men with classic hypogonadism and that drug labels should state that the efficacy and safety of testosterone products have not been established for age-related hypogonadism. In addition, because there is no evidence of laboratory testing before the initial testosterone prescription for some men, committee members recommended adding a statement to drug labels about the need to confirm low serum testosterone concentrations before initiating treatment'.

Effectively, the FDA has taken it upon themselves to define *testosterone deficiency* in terms of low testosterone and pulls the rug from under any physician who dares to disagree. They then strike a dangerous blow to the future of TRT by requiring manufacturers of testosterone products to band together to conduct a long-term controlled clinical trial to 'better determine the effects of testosterone therapy on cardiovascular outcomes among users'.

This, as the FDA probably well know, is a complete nonstarter for several reasons. Firstly, why should highly competitive pharmaceutical rivals making a wide variety of testosterone preparations pour millions of dollars into any one product and limit sales for up to ten years to come up with results which are unlikely to be more conclusive than the results already found in expensive controlled trials before marketing? It sounds like what will be described in politics as a filibuster, a meaningless exercise just to induce delay while patients badly needing treatment go untreated.

Also, the routine academic cry at the end of every publication of 'more research before we can routinely recommend this treatment' means that in fact, we want to sit on the fence and do nothing except award ourselves and our coworkers, big long-term research grants and continue to go to conferences in nice places indefinitely.

By contrast with this academic procrastination, let me give you an example of what can currently be achieved with testosterone treatment. With a couple of knowledgeable academic colleagues, I published a paper in a highly rated journal in the field after a year of writing and review by three referees who caused considerable revision of the paper. It was a review of clinical experience over twenty-five years using seven different forms of testosterone treatment at the three Centre for Men's Health in London, Manchester, and Edinburgh.[4] It was probably the biggest and longest such study in the world involving over 2,000 men, giving in total over 4,500 man-years of experience.

It clearly showed several original findings. It showed the diverse hormonal changes associated with each treatment, yet there was sustained relief of the characteristic symptoms with each of them. The treatment was safe and in fact beneficial to the prostate, as had been shown in a previous analysis of the findings, with no increase in either benign or malignant changes in the prostate as reported in a previous paper.[5] Neither were there any adverse changes in cardiovascular risk factors on the treatments. In fact, there were some beneficial changes in terms of significant reductions in cholesterol and blood pressure. The article also showed how the cost of treatment could be reduced to less than that of antidepressants, a most cheering and encouraging finding.

Intriguingly, it again showed that there was no relationship between testosterone levels before starting treatment and either symptoms of testosterone deficiency or the likelihood of a good response to treatment. It also showed that using pretreatment testosterone levels as cutoff points to decide which symptomatic cases should have the benefits of treatment resulted in over 90 percent of cases missing out.

You might have thought that the medical establishment might have welcomed this clarification of whom and how to give testosterone treatment as based on extensive experience of testosterone treatment, but not a bit of it. Immediately, the article, when reported in the popular press, was greeted by those who might be described as the usual suspects with the following damning criticisms:

1. Firstly, they made a concerted effort to rubbish the study by describing it as being 'below the normal standards of science' since it was not a double blind controlled trial. However, this response raised the question of whether it was ethical to conduct such a trial of a group of medications which you knew could immediately transform the lives of people suffering the clear symptoms of a life-wrecking disease which can easily, rapidly, and safely be reversed, as many short-term, more academically correct studies had shown over the last seventy years since testosterone first became available.

   Also, if the referees of a specialist journal in the field, after careful review, had decided it should be published, who were the critics to say it should not be and ignore twenty-five years of carefully documented clinical evidence?

2. The critics then went onto say that the authors were obviously unaware of the expert guidelines saying that testosterone treatment should only be prescribed according to the threshold values of testosterone that had been set in stone by international organizations setting the conditions rules for treatment.

My answer to that would be that testosterone values had been shown to be subject to up to 100 percent variation according to sampling and laboratory factors, as well as interpretation, and were totally unreliable as a basis for diagnosing testosterone deficiency.[6] If they were, I would not be arguing in favor of using clinical history and symptoms as basis for the diagnosis of testosterone deficiency. So over the years, I had spent many hours studying and comparing various guidelines and, on the subject of criteria for the diagnosis of testosterone deficiency, could place little or no faith in cutoff levels of testosterone.

Then of course, there are the factors in internal resistance to the action of any given level of testosterone, which I have described previously.

I know that modern, evidence-based scientific medicine much prefers laboratory values to questionnaires as for the diagnosis of disease, but there is loads of scientific evidence that this is not the situation in the diagnosis of testosterone deficiency. Unfortunately, there is no lab test that gives a reliable diagnosis of testosterone deficiency any more than there is a test for depression. Depressing, but that's the way it is.

3. Critics also say that the study was 'misleading and potentially dangerous'. Well, it is only misleading if you believe that the level of testosterone in the blood is the main arbiter of treatment and wish to argue against the principle of testosterone resistance and the variability of symptoms in relation to the level of testosterone, which was carefully explained in the article and carefully evidenced. It is curious that the very academics who say the treatment is dangerous are the ones who, twenty years ago, were proving it safety as a male contraceptive in doses two to three times higher than usually used for routine TRT.

    The same people will go on to give as an example of the dangers a rise in red blood cell numbers, called polycythemia, which occurred in one overdosed case treated with short-acting testosterone injections and not properly monitored. These injections are no longer used by any reputable expert in the field, precisely because they give a rollercoaster ride in symptoms rather than the smooth improvement that the daily treatments or long-lasting injections usually give.

4. Next up, the critics ignore the fact that the authors have moved on from calling the typical symptom complex the male menopause to the preferable and less-ageist term testosterone deficiency syndrome. They refer back to the thirty-year-old argument that unlike the abrupt drop in estrogens occurring about the age of fifty at the

menopause in women, there is only a 0.4 percent drop in testosterone in the age of thirty onwards. Mind you, that is an admitted 12 percent in what are average figures by age sixty, when, because of increasing testosterone resistance, this can make a critical difference to its action.

Also, there is the interesting fact that two studies, one in America[7] and one in Finland,[8] showing that overall testosterone levels in the male population are falling quite rapidly and alarmingly to the point where young men have the same levels as that of their twenty to thirty years older fathers. This may be due to increasing rates of obesity, scrotal warming in tighter trousers, environmental estrogens, and even pesticides. Whatever the causes, which may be multiple, both testosterone levels and sperm counts are falling in many countries till we have nearly reached a tipping point, where population numbers start to decrease.

Because the 0.4 percent is only an average figure and common factors in a man's life such as stress, alcohol, and increasing abdominal obesity, combined with decreasing fitness, can cause this drop to be greater and more rapid in the at least 20 percent of men over the age of fifty who develop the typical symptoms, slow decline in testosterone levels is a faulty argument even if routinely trotted out.

5. Then comes the argument that the main reason some older men have low testosterone levels is not the so-called manopause but underlying problems such as

obesity and age-related illnesses such as type 2 diabetes and heart failure. Heavy drinking, stress, depression, and medication—including certain painkillers—can also lower T levels. 'We men are hardwired to shut down testosterone levels when we are ill,' opponents explain. 'In these cases, it is the underlying problem which needs treatment, not the low testosterone levels.'

This is the chicken-and-egg argument. Is it the illness causing the low testosterone or the low testosterone causing the illness? Why not give testosterone and find out?

Well, except for the fact we have shown that it is not the level of testosterone which is the decisive factor in whether symptoms of testosterone deficiency develop and the illnesses quoted both lower testosterone levels and increase resistance to its action, saying that he won't need the help of testosterone treatment to overcome them seems faintly punitive and ridiculous.

6. Then comes the claim that the increasing use of testosterone treatment, as in America, where sales have increase by a factor of tenfold in the last ten years, must be due to disease-mongering rather than legitimate prescribing by doctors increasingly aware of true testosterone deficiency symptoms and the relief that TRT can provide. This is again based on making the diagnosis by the level of testosterone in the blood rather than on symptoms and their relief. Rigid application of a totally irrelevant test can be called disease denial, blatantly refusing to recognize testosterone deficiency

symptoms as a means of denying TRT to the millions of men needing it.

Twenty years ago, at a meeting on men's health, when asking one such denier why GPs were failing to treat these manifest symptoms, he asserted that GPs were the gatekeepers of the NHS and were charged with keeping the hordes of men who might demand treatment away from such a dangerous and, in his opinion, unnecessary therapeutic trial. I then replied that I thought in this case the GPs were slamming the gate in the faces of the men needing treatment. Not surprisingly, it didn't go down well.

7. Then they subtly play the outdated 'danger of prostate cancer' card, often with an advertisement for a prostate cancer charity. They suggest that TRT can increase PSA, which it may do in the early stages of treatment in severely testosterone-deficient men, while it remains in the normal range for many years of treatment afterward. Also, which they don't mention, it definitely does not increase prostate cancer risks, as a previous UKAS study, along with many others, has shown.[9]

8. Next, they routinely quote the faulty studies on TRT causing heart disease, which we have already demolished, but hey ho, on we go! Why muzzle the attack dogs?

9. Finally, they exaggerate the claims that even the most enthusiastic proponents of TRT may, but actually don't make to, say 'TRT is definitely not a cure-all'. 'What man of my age wouldn't want to put on muscle?' he asks.

'Who wouldn't want to be reborn?' It's the old panacea trick and quite unworthy of serious scientific debate.

So where do we go in the face of such implacable opposition by the academic establishment, the do-little doctors of this world who are rapidly becoming Dr Nos?

Firstly, we stick with our medical colleagues who are quietly getting on with high-quality research showing the benefits of TRT in a wide range of conditions, including diabetes,[10, 11, 12] obesity, metabolic syndrome,[13, 14, 15] and even Alzheimer's disease.[16]

Secondly, and probably more importantly, given the testosterone resistance of the medical establishment and providing authorities and their entrenched opposition to TRT, we must enlist the help of what I call the patient's voice. This is the vast number of men experiencing the typical symptoms of testosterone deficiency as measured by the AMS questionnaire and comparing it with the experience of the relatively few men who have managed to get treatment for these symptoms.

This was the experience of over 10,000 men, mainly from the UK (70 percent) and USA (10 percent), who filled in the AMS questionnaire online on three different UK-based websites in 2011.[17] Among them, 80 percent had moderate or severe scores suggesting that they would be likely to benefit from TRT. The average age of these men was fifty-two, with many cases in their forties, an age when the diagnosis of late-onset hypogonadism was not generally considered. Other possible contributory factors to the high testosterone deficiency scores reported were obesity (29 percent), alcohol (17.3 percent), testicular problems such as mumps orchitis (11.4 percent), prostate problems (5.6 percent), urinary infection (5.2 percent), and diabetes (5.7 percent).

From this large-scale study it was concluded that in this self-selected international sample of men, there was a very high prevalence of scores which would warrant a therapeutic trial of testosterone treatment. The study suggests that there are large numbers of men in the community whose testosterone deficiency is neither being diagnosed nor treated. The large number of men responding to the questionnaire and giving high scores has not abated since that study was carried out, and a follow-up is planned to see what has happened to these very largely untreated men and increase awareness of their unsolved problem.

Thirdly, given the vast number of untreated men round the world likely to be suffering the symptoms and side effects of testosterone deficiency, we have to acknowledge that it doesn't take a high powered consultant andrologist, endocrinologist or urologist to diagnose and treat the condition. A well trained general practitioner willing to follow the simple guidelines for diagnosing testosterone deficiency and monitoring the patient's progress can easily use the treatment in the majority of cases. In the process they can enjoy the satisfaction of often giving the man a new lease of healthy life.

Let's just encourage those willing to look at the wide-ranging but usually totally ignored evidence that TRT can help in the prevention and treatment of the following conditions:

1. Symptoms of testosterone deficiency

2. Erectile dysfunction

3. Diabetes and its complications

4. Cardiovascular disease and preventing heart failure

5. Peripheral vascular disease and preventing gangrene

6. Some stages of prostate cancer

7. AIDS (HIV infections)

8. Depression

9. Early Alzheimer's disease

10. Parkinson's disease

11. Multiple sclerosis

12. Trauma to the head and spinal cord

13. Osteoporosis

14. Frailty of aging

15. Prolongation of life

Of course, it's not a panacea, but given the above it would seem to be as good a candidate as any current drug can claim to be. Sometimes, this term is taken to mean a cure for a large, multifaceted problem, which, in the case of metabolic syndrome, with its combination of diabetes, lipid disturbances, and hypertension, it certainly seems to come close to.

Of course, skeptics will find studies that appear to deny its benefit in these conditions, but I will suggest that the weight of evidence is strongly in its favor.   You are invited to look up reference libraries such as PubMed, and decide for yourself where the balance of evidence lies in any or all these conditions that interest you.

To finish on a hopeful note in this turbulent tale of the fight for testosterone treatment, at a meeting in October 2015 of the International Society for the Study of the Aging Male (ISSAM), there was a consensus conference on testosterone deficiency and its treatment, chaired by Prof. Abe Morgentaler, a urologist from Boston, and Prof. Michael Zitzman, an endocrinologist from München in Germany. The eighteen strong groups of international experts debated and agreed on the following resolutions:

1. Testosterone deficiency (TD) is a well-established, significant medical condition that negatively affects male sexuality, reproduction, and quality of life.

2. Symptoms and signs of TD occur as a result of low levels of testosterone and may benefit from treatment regardless if there is an underlying etiology.

3. TD is a global public health concern.

4. Testosterone therapy for men with TD is effective, rational, and evidence-based.

5. There is no T concentration that reliably distinguishes those who will respond to treatment from those who will not.

6. There is no scientific basis for recommendations against the use of T therapy in men over sixty-five years.

7. The evidence does not support increased risks of cardiovascular events with T therapy.

8. The evidence does not support increased risk of prostate cancer with T therapy.

9. Current evidence supports a major research initiative to explore possible benefits of T therapy for cardiometabolic disease.

The consensus agreement on these nine key points by these world experts, none of whom were influenced by pharmaceutical company sponsorship, were put forward to a press conference the same afternoon and gave great encouragement for the over 300 conference delegates who were coming to hear the latest news on TRT, its safety, and its effectiveness.

It seems only by the mobilization of public opinion in favor of testosterone treatment, and the gradual overcoming of establishment resistance to the treatment by the already massive accumulation of favorable clinical evidence that TRT will come to be seen as great an advance in preventive and therapeutic medicine for the twenty-first century as HRT was for women in the twentieth century. It can then achieve proper recognition as being the 'Men's Health Hormone'

This is best seen as the intended prolongation of healthy life so that men can live their life in square wave form like alkaline batteries going full charge to the end (figure 1)!

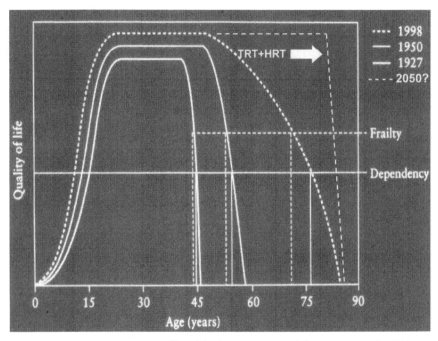

Figure 1. Gains in years of healthy living expected from TRT and HRT

References for Chapter 7

[1] M. Carruthers, T. T. Trinick, and M. J. Wheeler, 'The Validity of Androgen Assays', *Aging Male*, 10/3 (2007), 165–172.

[2] M. Carruthers, P. J. Cathcart, and M. R. Feneley, 'Evolution of Testosterone Treatment over 25 Years: Symptom Responses, Endocrine Profiles and Cardiovascular Changes', *Aging Male* (2015).

[3] C. P. Nguyen, M. S. Hirsch, D. Moeny, S. Kaul, M. Mohamoud, and H. V. Joffe, 'Testosterone and Age-Related Hypogonadism—FDA Concerns', *New England Journal of Medicine*, 373/8 (2015), 689–691.

[4] M. Carruthers, P. J. Cathcart, and M. R. Feneley, 'Evolution of Testosterone Treatment over 25 Years: Symptom Responses, Endocrine Profiles and Cardiovascular Changes', *Aging Male* (2015).

[5] M. R. Feneley and M. Carruthers, 'Is Testosterone Treatment Good for the Prostate? Study of Safety During Long-Term Treatment', *Journal of Sexual Medicine*, 9/8 (2012), 2,138–2,149.

[6] M. Carruthers, T. R. Trinick, and M. J. Wheeler, 'The Validity of Androgen Assays', *Aging Male*, 10/3 (2007), 165–172.

[7] T. G. Travison, A. B. Araujo, A. B. O'Donnell, V. Kupelian, and J. B. McKinlay, 'A Population-Level Decline in Serum Testosterone Levels in American Men', *Journal of Clinical Endocrinology and Metabolism*, 92/1 (2007), 196–202.

[8] A. Perheentupa, J. Mäkinen, T. Laatikainen, M. Vierula, N. E. Skakkebaek, A. M. Andersson, et al., 'A cohort effect on serum testosterone levels in Finnish men', *European journal of*

endocrinology / European Federation of Endocrine Societies, 168/2 (2013), 227–233.

[9.] M. R. Feneley and M. Carruthers, 'Is Testosterone Treatment Good for the Prostate? Study of Safety During Long-Term Treatment', *Journal of Sexual Medicine*, 9/8 (2012), 2,138–2,149.

[10.] T. H. Jones, 'Testosterone, Insulin Resistance and Type 2 Diabetes', *Journal of Endocrinology, Metabolism and Diabetes of South Africa*, 19/1 (2014), 22–24.

[11.] P. M. Rao, D. M. Kelly, and T. H. Jones, 'Testosterone and Insulin Resistance in the Metabolic Syndrome and T2DM in Men', *Nature Reviews Endocrinology*, 9/8 (2013), 479–493.

[12.] V. Muraleedharan, H. Marsh, D. Kapoor, K. S. Channer, and T. H. Jones, 'Testosterone Deficiency Is Associated with Increased Risk of Mortality and Testosterone Replacement Improves Survival in Men with Type 2 Diabetes', *European Journal Endocrinology*, 169/6 (2013), 725–733.

[13.] F. Saad, 'The Emancipation of Testosterone from Niche Hormone to Multisystem Player', *Asian Journal of Andrology*, 17/1 (2015), 58–60.

[14.] A. Yassin, D. J. Yassin, P. G. Hammerer, G. Doros, and F. Saad, 'Long-Term Testosterone Treatment Has Favourable Effects in Obese Hypogonadal Men on Body Weight and Prostate Health Parameters', *European Urology* Supplements, 13/1 (2014), e780.

[15.] F. Saad, G. Doros, A. Haider, and A. Traish, 'Obese Hypogonadal Men Benefit from Long-Term Testosterone Treatment with Testosterone Undecanoate Injections in Multiple Ways', *Journal of Sexual* Medicine, 10 (2013), 257–258.

16. P. R. Asih, E. J. Wahjoepramono, V. Aniwiyanti, L. K. Wijaya, K. De Ruyck, K. Taddei, et al., 'Testosterone Replacement Therapy in Older Male Subjective Memory Complainers: Double-Blind Randomized Crossover Placebo-Controlled Clinical Trial of Physiological Assessment and Safety', *CNS and Neurological Disorders—Drug Targets*, 14/5 (2015), 576–586.

17. T. R. Trinick, M. R. Feneley, H. Welford, and M. Carruthers, 'International Web Survey Shows High Prevalence of Symptomatic Testosterone Deficiency in Men', *Aging Male*, 14/1 (2011), 10–15.

Aging Males' Symptoms questionnarie

Aging Males' Symptoms (AMS) questionnaire. Taken from Lunenfeld B, Gooren L, eds. *Textbook of Men's Health*. London: Parthenon Publishing, 2002:34

Which of the following symptoms apply to you at this time? Please, mark the appropriate box for each symptom. For symptoms that do not apply, please mark "none".

	Symptoms				
Score =	none 1	mild 2	moderate 3	severe 4	extremely severe 5
1. Decline in your feeling of general well-being (general state of health, subjective feeling)	☐	☐	☐	☐	☐
2. Joint pain and muscular ache (lower back pain, joint pain, pain in a limb, general back ache)	☐	☐	☐	☐	☐
3. Excessive sweating (unexpected/sudden episodes of sweating, hot flushes independent of strain)	☐	☐	☐	☐	☐
4. Sleep problems (difficulty in falling asleep, difficulty in sleeping through, waking up early and feeling tired, poor sleep, sleeplessness)	☐	☐	☐	☐	☐
5. Increased need for sleep, often feeling tired	☐	☐	☐	☐	☐
6. Irritability (feeling aggressive, easily upset about little things, moody)	☐	☐	☐	☐	☐
7. Nervousness (inner tension, restlessness, feeling fidgety)	☐	☐	☐	☐	☐
8. Anxiety (feeling panicky)	☐	☐	☐	☐	☐
9. Physical exhaustion / lacking vitality (general decrease in performance, reduced activity, lacking interest in leisure activities, feeling of getting less done, of achieving less, of having to force oneself to undertake activities)	☐	☐	☐	☐	☐
10. Decrease in muscular strength (feeling of weakness)	☐	☐	☐	☐	☐
11. Depressive mood (feeling down, sad, on the verge of tears, lack of drive, mood swings, feeling nothing is of any use)	☐	☐	☐	☐	☐
12. Feeling that you have passed your peak	☐	☐	☐	☐	☐
13. Feeling burnt out, having hit rock-bottom	☐	☐	☐	☐	☐
14. Decrease in beard growth	☐	☐	☐	☐	☐
15. Decrease in ability/frequency to perform sexually	☐	☐	☐	☐	☐
16. Decrease in the number of morning erections	☐	☐	☐	☐	☐
17. Decrease in sexual desire/libido (lacking pleasure in sex, lacking desire for sexual intercourse)	☐	☐	☐	☐	☐

Likelihood of Testosterone Deficiency Syndrome according to total sum of all subscales:

17-26 : Unlikely   27-36 : Little   37-49 : Moderate   50 or more : Severe

Other Books by Professor Carruthers

1. *The Western Way of Death: Stress, Tension and Heart Disease*, 1973

2. *Fats on Trial*, 1975

3. *Real Health: The Ill Effects of Stress and Their Prevention*, 1980

4. *F/40: Fitness on Forty Minutes a Week*, 1978

5. *Male Menopause: Restoring Vitality and Virility*, 1996

6. *Maximising Manhood: Beating the Male Menopause*, 1997

7. *The Testosterone Revolution: Rediscover Your Energy and Overcome the Symptoms of the Male Menopause*, 2001

8. *ADAM: Androgen Deficiency in the Adult Male—Causes, Diagnosis, and Treatment*, 2004

Published Papers on Testosterone (Refereed)

1. M. Carruthers, 'HRT for the Aging Male: A Clinical Study in 1,000 Men', *The Aging Male*, 1/1 (1998), 34.

2. M. Carruthers, 'Androgen Deficiency in the Aging Male (ADAM): A Multilevel and Multinational Crisis', *The Aging Male*, 14/3 (2000), 58.

3. M. Carruthers, 'More Effective Testosterone Treatment: Combination with Sildenafil and Danazol', *The Aging Male*, 3/1 (2000), 16.

4. M. Carruthers, 'A Multifactorial Approach to Understanding Andropause', *Journal of Sexual and Reproductive Medicine*, 1/2 (2001), 69–74.

5. M. Carruthers, 'The Safety of Long-Term Testosterone Treatment', *The Aging Male*, 4/4 (2002), 255.

6. M. Carruthers, 'The Diagnosis of Androgen Deficiency', *The Aging Male*, 4/4 (2002), 254.

7. M. Carruthers, 'Androgens and the Blood/Brain Barrier', *Andrologia*, 36/3 (2004), 212–213.

8. M. Carruthers and T. R. Trinick, 'The Validity of Androgen Assays', *The Aging Male*, 10/3 (2004), 165.

9. M. R. Feneley and M. Carruther, 'PSA Monitoring during Testosterone Replacement Therapy: Low Long-Term Risk of Prostate Cancer with Improved Opportunity for Cure', *Andrologia*, 36/4 (2004), 212.

10. K. A. Bates, A. R. Harvey, M. Carruthers, and R. N. Martins, 'Androgens, Andropause and Neurodegeneration: Exploring the Link between Steroidogenesis, Androgens and Alzheimer's Disease', *Cellular and Molecular Life Sciences*, 62/3 (2005), 281–292.

11. M. Carruthers, 'Transdermal Testosterone Treatments', *JEAMM*, 1/2 (2005), 24–27.

12. M. Carruthers, 'An Androgen Resistance Syndrome (ARS) in the Adult Male?', *The Aging Male*, 9/1 (2006), 5.

13. M. R. Feneley and M. E. Carruthers, 'Androgens: The Prostate and Safety of Testosterone Treatment', *The Aging Male*, 9/1 (2006), 4.

14. M. Carruthers, T. R. Trinick, and M. J. Wheeler, 'The Validity of Androgen Assays', *The Aging Male*, 10/3 (2007), 165–172.

15. M. Carruthers, 'The Paradox Dividing Testosterone Deficiency Symptoms and Androgen Assays: A Closer Look at the Cellular and Molecular Mechanisms of Androgen Action', *Journal of Sexual Medicine*, 5/4 (2008), 998–1,012.

16. M. Carruthers, T. R. Trinick, E. Jankowska, and A. M. Traish, 'Are the Adverse Effects of Glitazones Linked to Induced Testosterone Deficiency?', *Cardiovascular Diabetology*, 7 (2008), 30.

17. E. J. Wahjoepramono, L. K. Wijaya, K. Taddei, G. Martins, M. Howard, R. K. de, et al., 'Distinct Effects of Testosterone on Plasma and Cerebrospinal Fluid Amyloid-Beta Levels', *Journal of Alzheimer's Disease*, 15/1 (2008), 129–137.

18. M. Carruthers, 'Time for International Action on Treating Testosterone Deficiency Syndrome', *The Aging Male*, 12/1 (2009), 21–28.

19. M. Carruthers and M. R. Feneley, 'Endocrine Changes in Different Forms of Long-Term Testosterone Treatment: The UK Androgen Study (UKAS)', *Journal of Sexual Medicine* (2011).

20. M. Carruthers, 'Sex Steroids and Alzheimer's Disease (invited paper)', *Journal of Aging Research* (2011).

21. M. Carruthers, 'The Concept of Androgen Resistance in the Testosterone Deficiency Syndrome', *Journal of*

Reproductive Medicine and Endocrinology, 8/3 (2011), 201–202.

22. M. R. Feneley and M. Carruthers, 'Is Testosterone Treatment Good for the Prostate? Study of Safety During Long-Term Treatment', *Journal of Reproductive Medicine and Endocrinology*, 8/3 (2011), 206.

23. T. R. Trinick, M. R. Feneley, H. Welford, and M. Carruthers, 'International Web Survey Shows High Prevalence of Symptomatic Testosterone Deficiency in Men', *The Aging Male*, 14/1 (2011), 10–15.

24. M. Carruthers, 'Testosterone Deficiency Syndrome: Cellular and Molecular Mechanism of Action', *Current Aging Science*, 6/1 (2013), 115–124.

25. R. Martins and M. Carruthers, 'Testosterone as the Missing Link between Pesticides, Alzheimer's Disease, and Parkinson's Disease', *JAMA Neurology*, 71/9 (2014), 1,189–1,190.

26. P. R. Asih, E. J. Wahjoepramono, V. Aniwiyanti, L. K. Wijaya, K. De Ruyck, K. Taddei, et al., 'Testosterone Replacement Therapy in Older Male Subjective Memory Complainers: Double-Blind Randomized Crossover Placebo-Controlled Clinical Trial of Physiological Assessment and Safety', *CNS and Neurological Disorders—Drug Targets*, 14/5 (2015), 576–586.

27. M. Carruthers, P. J. Cathcart, and M. R. Feneley, 'Evolution of Testosterone Treatment over 25 Years: Symptom Responses, Endocrine Profiles and Cardiovascular Changes', *The Aging Male*, 18/4 (2015), 217–227.

Index